THE
MIRACLE
OF
VINEGAR

To my gorgeous sons Rory and Ewan for their enduring patience, boundless creativity and sharing their brilliant recipe ideas with me.

— *Aggie*

Thanks to my mum for my culinary drive, to Kev for always tasting everything I've made (no matter what time of day) and to the rest of my family for their support.

— *Emma*

THE MIRACLE OF VINEGAR

AGGIE MACKENZIE
& EMMA MARSDEN

HQ
An imprint of HarperCollins*Publishers* Ltd
1 London Bridge Street
London SE1 9GF

www.harpercollins.co.uk

HarperCollins*Publishers*
Macken House, 39/40 Mayor Street Upper,
Dublin 1, D01 C9W8, Ireland

This edition 2023

2

First published in Great Britain by
HQ, an imprint of HarperCollins*Publishers* Ltd 2019

HB ISBN: 978-0-00-831057-8
PB ISBN: 978-0-00-852560-6

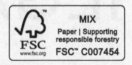

MIX
Paper | Supporting
responsible forestry
FSC™ C007454
FSC
www.fsc.org

This book is produced from independently certified FSC™ paper
to ensure responsible forest management.

For more information visit: www.harpercollins.co.uk/green

Printed and Bound in the UK using 100% Renewable Electricity at
CPI Group (UK) Ltd, Croydon, CR0 4YY

CONTENTS

CONTENTS

INTRODUCTION

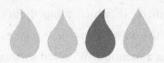

Vinegar first came into my working life while I was at *Good Housekeeping* magazine in the early 1990s. I was director of the Institute and in this role I oversaw both the consumer testing and cookery departments. Each year, the January issue of the magazine carried a 'Stains Special'… and vinegar always featured prominently.

When, in 2002, I was asked to do a screen test for a new television programme about cleaning, I drew on my *GH* experience and rattled off a list of all the kooky remedies I had picked up over the years, and again vinegar enjoyed multiple name-checks.

I passed the screen test, got the TV gig and co-presented *How Clean is Your House?* on Channel 4 from 2003 to 2009. My co-presenter and I generally used old-fashioned, inexpensive and homespun remedies for clean-ups – and very soon vinegar became the star of the show.

I am currently, about once a month, the 'Midnight Expert' guest on the BBC Radio 5 Live Phil Williams show. People call in and text between midnight and 1am with their cleaning quandaries – it's strange but true, there is never any shortage of queries, even at that late hour. So often have I named vinegar as the solution to removing a stain that Phil, a good while back, instigated 'Aggie's Vinegar Bingo', in which a big shout-out goes to the caller who, during the on-air hour, nails the nearest time to the V-word first getting a mention. Who knew vinegar could create so much buzz?

Vinegar is said to have been discovered by accident around 10,000 years ago, and it can be made from almost any fermentable item – such as wine, apples, pears, grapes, berries, beer and potatoes.

For over 2000 years, vinegar has been used to flavour and preserve foods, heal wounds and fight infections – as well as clean surfaces. There is some evidence that vinegar added to one's diet will reduce the glucose response to a carbohydrate load both in healthy adults and in sufferers of diabetes. It has also been suggested that drinking a little vinegar each day is useful as a dietary aid because it imparts a feeling of fullness. Since I began working on this book I have been drinking two tablespoons of organic cider vinegar with a tiny squeeze of honey every morning. Who knows whether it's doing me any good, but I am sure it won't be doing me much harm either.

Both my sons are chefs in leading London restaurants and often use specialist vinegars for finishing dishes. Through them I have learned what a difference it can make and how to use it judiciously in my cooking.

It seemed natural that I should put my head together with that of my friend and former cookery editor colleague at *Good Housekeeping*, Emma Marsden, to come up with a book that combines my cleaning-with-vinegar expertise and her extensive culinary knowledge. Here is our – we hope – useful collection of tips, plus recipes that are, without exception, exciting, innovative and, importantly, straightforward. We hope you'll enjoy them, together with beauty remedies and health hints – all using this humble yet important liquid in its many and various forms.

Aggie MacKenzie

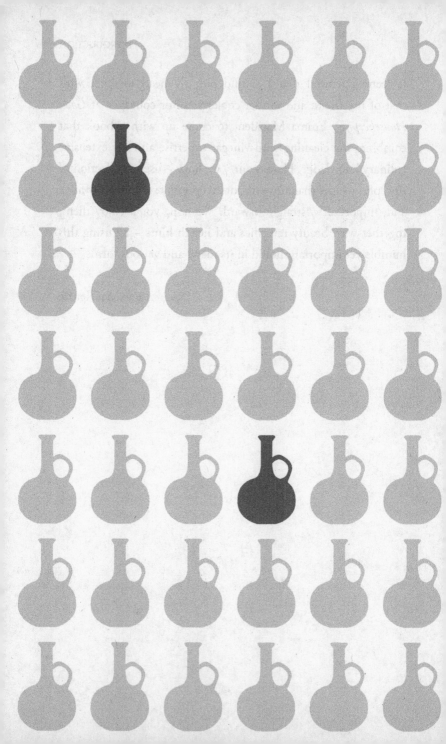

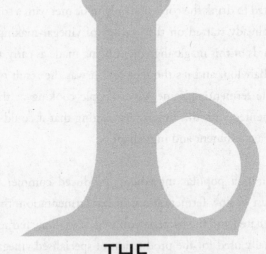

THE
HISTORY
OF
VINEGAR

The word vinegar comes from the French *vin aigre,* translated as sour wine, which accurately describes it. If you've ever left the dregs of an open bottle of wine for a few days and then attempted to drink the contents, only to be met with a sour taste, you've already started on the journey of vinegar-making. There are records of this magic ingredient being made as early as 5,000 BC in Babylon, and it's thought that it was the result of a slip-up while fermenting some wine. People cooking at that time experimented with this liquor, discovering that it could be used as both a condiment and ingredient.

Today it is a popular ingredient, produced commercially by either fast or slow fermentation. In fast fermentation, the liquid is oxygenated and the bacteria culture added. Slow fermentation is generally used for the production of specialised vinegars used in cooking; the culture of acetic acid bacteria grows on the surface of the liquid and fermentation evolves gradually over weeks or months and allows for the formation of a harmless slime made up of yeast and acetic acid bacteria, also known as the vinegar mother.

As history has already told, you can by all means leave a bottle of wine open – covered with a cloth that lets in air but not fruit flies – and eventually it will turn into vinegar. It may take months, though, so if you want to speed up the process and guarantee a result, here are a few pointers.

Firstly, vinegar is like sourdough and yogurt, in that it's good to have some kind of starter to begin with. With sourdough it's a leaven to add to flour and water; with yogurt it's a couple of tablespoons of yogurt to add to milk that's then heated. For vinegar, it's some unpasteurised vinegar with the mother to start the process. These bottles are labelled clearly and you can buy them online and in supermarkets and delis.

Secondly, you need time. The mixture of wine and a vinegar mother won't turn into vinegar overnight. You need a dark cupboard and the patience to wait for the mixture to ferment and the bacteria from the vinegar mother to turn the alcohol into acetic acid.

Thirdly, you need oxygen from the air, so use a wide-mouthed jar or ceramic pot and cover it with muslin or cheesecloth so the oxygen can get in but bugs can't.

Whether you're making wine or beer vinegar (see pages 13–17), the basic recipe is much the same. Pour 400ml red wine or beer into a large open-mouthed jar (either ceramic or glass) then pour 200ml unpasteurised cider vinegar with the mother into the jar, too. Cover with a muslin or cheesecloth square and secure with a band. Label and store in a cool dark place for at least one month. It may take longer depending on conditions, but just keep tasting as you go. Some vinegar will naturally evaporate so, depending on how long it takes for the vinegar to brew, you'll get around 400ml to use. You may find that a jelly-like substance forms in the liquid – don't bin this, lift it out and transfer to another sterilised jar and use it to make another batch of vinegar with some of the unpasteurised liquor you've just fermented.

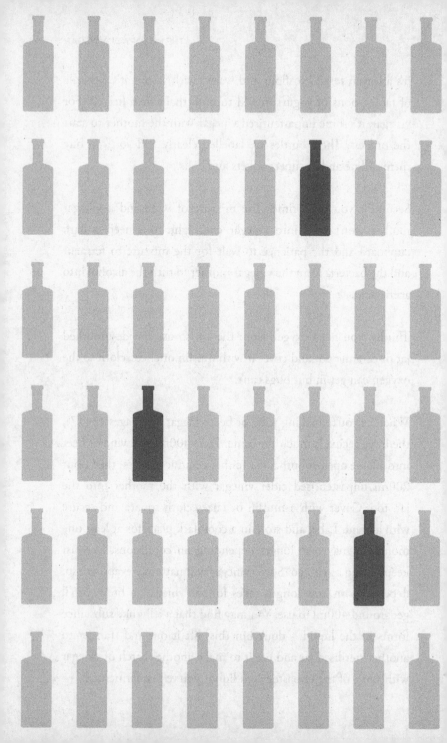

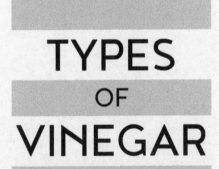

TYPES
OF
VINEGAR

With such an array of vinegars available, it can be bewildering to know which to choose – you don't want to use an expensive sherry vinegar to clean your windows, nor might you want to add a brash distilled malt to a casserole.

The most common vinegars produced in this country are malt (the brown stuff you put on fish and chips) and distilled malt (the clear type used in cleaning and food preserving).

With wine and sherry vinegars, the quality of the base alcohol used has a direct bearing on how good the vinegar will taste. A decent wine vinegar will be aged for a number of years in wooden casks, which imbues complex and mellow tones.

Balsamic is in a class of its own: look for the terms *tradizionale* and DOC. Cheap versions will have been coloured and flavoured with caramel and won't have the authentic flavour balance.

The inclusion of a good wine or sherry vinegar in a soup or stew can often reduce the amount of salt you would normally use. It can also help you cut the amount of fat required in a recipe because vinegar is a great balancer of flavours, thus lessening the need for as much cream, butter or oil. It's worth experimenting with different types – you'll soon find out what best suits you. As you read through the descriptions of the most popular vinegars here, we're sure you'll identify one or two that will match your palate and style of cooking.

WHICH VINEGAR WHEN?

BALSAMIC VINEGAR

The more you pay, the better the quality. Look for a vinegar that has been aged for several years and contains more grape must than wine vinegar – it will have a syrupy consistency and a fabulous depth of flavour. Save your posh one to use with figs and strawberries.

• • •

BEER VINEGAR

No surprises here – the base of this is beer, but it is brewed with a vinegar mother to achieve the acidity. Flavours vary from lighter styles to dark rich notes depending on which ale is used.

• • •

CHINESE VINEGAR

The main ingredients here are the same as rice vinegar, sometimes with added spice, and the colour comes from an additive. Good for marinades and stir-fries.

CIDER VINEGAR

Also known as apple cider vinegar. Similar to a sharp, acidic flat cider with a vinegary, apple-y aftertaste. Next time you're cooking pork chops, add a knob of butter to the pan juices plus a splash of this for a simple sauce. Or try this in a quick tuna pâté (see page 118). It also has some digestive benefits (see page 61).

• • •

DISTILLED MALT VINEGAR

This is produced by the distillation of malt, which gives a clear, colourless vinegar. Inexpensive; used mainly in pickling and preserving, and also for cleaning.

• • •

HONEY VINEGAR

Sharp and bright with no hint of sweetness. It has a strong kick, so use it sparingly. Good with the Chocolate Sharing Mousse on page 146.

• • •

MALT VINEGAR

Made from barley and dark brown in colour. It has a very sharp taste; it is traditionally sprinkled over fish and chips, but it's also really useful when making big batches of pickles or chutneys as it's inexpensive.

• • •

MOSCATEL VINEGAR

Sweet and raisin-y, with hints of honey and florals. If this is used in a dressing, reduce the suggested sugar quantity so as not to overdo the sweetness. Good with a soft, creamy blue cheese such as Gorgonzola dolce or Beauvale. For a new twist, use in the classic dressing for oysters – *sauce mignonette* (see page 130).

• • •

RASPBERRY VINEGAR

Bright pink with a thick consistency and a predominant fruity taste with a tart edge. Keep it for salad dressings and try it in the recipes on pages 100–1.

• • •

RED WINE VINEGAR

It's really worth pushing the boat out with this type of vinegar and looking for a particular grape, such as Merlot or Cabernet Sauvignon, as the flavour of these is incomparable. Some specialist red wine vinegars have been mixed with grape juice, which softens the sharpness, and are good for splashing into a dish of dark fruits. Or use them for finishing off a game dish. A basic red wine vinegar is fine for everyday dressings, but when you want a subtle sharpness with complex flavours, you do need to shell out for something a little more special. A good-quality red wine vinegar will have a well-rounded flavour that's tangy rather than acidic, and will also be less likely to cause acid reflux or heartburn in those prone to it.

• • •

RICE VINEGAR

This is made from rice and water, which are left to brew and then sometimes flavoured with salt. Useful for quick pickles (eg radish and cucumber) or for splashing over stir-fries.

• • •

SHERRY VINEGAR

Like sherry itself, from Fino to PX there's a huge range of flavours for this vinegar – and again, the more you spend, the more complex the character. Some makes have colour added, so check the bottle before you buy. A basic one is good added to gravies, or use it to cut through a fatty sausage – see tip on page 91 or the couscous salad on page 113. The PX vinegar is sweetish and smooth and works well with dark fruits such as blackberries.

• • •

VERJUS

Not strictly a vinegar, but it is often used in the same way to finish off recipes or added to pan sauces. It's made by pressing unripened green grapes and has a raisin-y/apple-y aroma and taste. Also good with summer fruits – see Peaches with Verjus and Rosemary on page 144 – and salads that feature toasted nuts and cheeses. It's not as sharp as most vinegars, so it allows other ingredients to sing rather than be swamped.

• • •

WHITE WINE VINEGAR

The go-to for a light salad dressing when you need a touch of acidity – use one-part vinegar to three-parts mild olive oil. You can also use it to make a shallot pickle to go with a curry as on page 94.

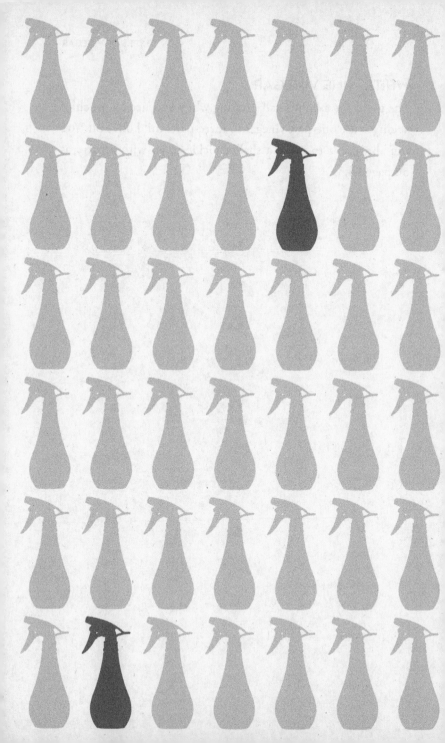

CLEANING
TIPS

A large Norwegian study widely publicised in the UK at the beginning of 2018 showed that regular use of cleaning sprays has a negative impact on lung health — similar to smoking 20 cigarettes a day over 10 to 20 years.

Vinegar, on the other hand, is biodegradable and provides a hostile environment for many types of germs. What makes it such a good cleaning agent? Acidity. Shop-bought distilled malt vinegar (the clear stuff) contains around 5% acetic acid and 95% water — fine for most general cleaning.

Vinegar is great for cutting through soap scum and limescale on shower glass, grease on cooker tops, and it'll strip wax build-up from a wooden floor. There's almost no end to the multitude of types of dreck it can conquer. (But don't use it on marble because it will mark the soft stone.)

You might want to vary the dilution depending on the task: you could use neat vinegar for mould on grouting or to disinfect a chopping board, whereas a 50:50 solution with water will work for general wiping down. A quick spritz of this mix will neutralise kitchen and bathroom smells.

Because it's natural, it's great for outdoor jobs such as wiping down patio furniture, cleaning exterior windows... and even getting rid of weeds!

KITCHEN

LIMESCALE ON TAPS

No need to spend your hard-earned cash on specialist products – much better to use bog-standard distilled malt vinegar (the clear, colourless stuff) instead. For ordinary chrome taps (don't use this on special finishes, it might be too strong and ruin your bespoke surface), soak a few sheets of kitchen paper with the vinegar, wrap these around the taps and cover with a plastic bag. Secure the lot with an elastic band so that the vinegar stays in contact with the taps and does its work. Leave on overnight, then the next morning, the scale should lift off fairly easily – just wipe it with a cloth. If it's really thick and annoyingly stubborn, repeat the process. You can take off any remaining bits of scale with a plastic scourer.

• • •

DESCALE YOUR KETTLE

If you live in a hard-water area you'll definitely have limescale, and the build-up of this is one of the main reasons why electric kettles meet their death. When the metal element gets coated with scale, this stops the heat getting into the water as efficiently, which can cause overheating (which will shorten the kettle's life). Stop this happening by descaling the kettle about once a month: fill it with half water and half clear vinegar – make sure it comes up over the scale line – and bring it to the boil. Switch off and leave overnight. Please note – it is really important to use *clear* vinegar for this; if you use the brown malt variety, the liquid inside the kettle will massively expand and erupt and you'll have a vinegary water mess all over the floor (this happened to me). Empty the kettle, rinse, refill and reboil a couple more times with plain water until every last trace of vinegariness has gone. If the scale is really bad and it's not all gone, repeat the process. If there are bits of scale around the rim, where the vinegar doesn't quite reach, gently rub around here with an emery board and it'll come off easily.

Next time you buy a kettle, get one with a built-in water filter. It'll improve the taste of your tea, get rid of scum and help reduce the amount of limescale build-up. Other things you can do are empty and rinse before refilling with fresh water each time you boil (this helps to get rid of loose scale), boil only as much water as you need, pour away any surplus water before it cools down, and empty the kettle before you go to bed.

• • •

ANYONE FOR SCALE-FREE COFFEE?
If your electric coffee maker has become a bit grotty and scale-bound, add a 50:50 ratio of clear vinegar and tap water to the water chamber and run the machine through a cycle, *sans* coffee.

Repeat this a couple more times, just with plain water. Some coffee-machine makers want you to use their own descalers, so check the instructions first to see if that's the case (it could affect the warranty if anything went wrong).

• • •

DEODORISE YOUR DISHWASHER

If your machine has suddenly developed a nasty whiff, first remove and wash the filter in hot soapy water, then check the spray arms for any bits of food and clean them, too. If you've never done this (which is perhaps the reason why you may have one or two problems), check the machine's manual to find out how to do it – it's really easy, and it's a good idea to do this weekly. Also, take a wodge of kitchen paper along the gap where the bottom of the door meets the base of the machine – you might get a shock at the amount of rotting dreck lurking there. Once you've done those bits, throw a cup of clear vinegar into the machine and run an empty cycle – this is great for keeping the pipes clear of grease and limescale.

• • •

BRING A SHINE TO YOUR FLOOR TILES

A soap-based cleaner can leave a tiled floor cloudy and dull, so to get that shiny finish, use a solution of mainly warm water with a good slug of clear vinegar. Make sure your mophead is made of microfibre (it cleans way more effectively, and most can be washed in the machine. There is no point in 'cleaning' a floor with a filthy mop).

• • •

BLOCKED SINK?

Before you call out an emergency plumber or spend a small fortune on environmentally unfriendly products, try this. Mix together 200g coarse salt and 100g bicarbonate of soda and pour it down the drain. Follow this with a cup of any type of vinegar plus a kettle full of boiling water. You'll witness a mini-explosion in your sink, but this is good – it'll help clear the blockage. Often (if the pipes are blocked with some solidified fat, for instance) this'll do the trick.

But don't wait until the kitchen sink gets blocked – treat your waste pipe to a monthly clear-out with a handful of bicarbonate of soda plus a cup of vinegar. Leave it to fizz for a minute or two, then follow through with a kettle of boiling water.

• • •

HARD-TO-GET-TO STAINS

To shift stubborn marks from a narrow-mouthed glass container (such as a decanter), mix 200–300ml warm water with the same of vinegar (any type) and pour it in. Add a handful of sand or uncooked rice, give it a good few swirls for around 30 seconds, then leave to stand for about an hour before pouring the mix away (but not down your sink or loo). Rinse well and the glass will sparkle like new.

• • •

SOMETHING SMELL FISHY?

If you've cooked fish and it's left a bad smell in the pan, half fill it with hot water plus a couple of tablespoons of clear vinegar, bring to the boil and simmer for 15 minutes. You might want to open a window to avoid being overpowered by the smell of vinegar!

•••

REFRESH YOUR MICROWAVE

Put a good slug of clear vinegar into a bowl of very hot water and heat in the microwave on High for around five minutes. The acidic steam will pass through the vents and loosen any food particles clinging to the sides. It'll now be easy to wipe clean with a damp cloth.

•••

A GRILLE'S BEST FRIEND

The metal grilles in a cooker hood get greasy very quickly, particularly if you're a fan of the frying pan. Most grilles nowadays are designed to go into the dishwasher, but if yours isn't one of those, give it a good soak overnight in a sink full of hot water with a cup each of clear vinegar and washing soda crystals. If your grilles won't easily fit into the sink, the bath is a good alternative (but first line the bottom with a large towel to avoid scratches to the surface). Afterwards, rinse the grille well and towel dry before putting it back into the hood.

•••

STEEL THE SHOW

If your stainless-steel sink has lost its shine or is covered with rusty stains, squirt a bit of washing-up liquid over the surface then scrub with a dampened pot scourer. Rinse and wipe down with a cloth dipped in clear vinegar then buff dry with either scrunched-up kitchen paper or newspaper. You'll need sunglasses to admire the shine.

•••

CUPBOARD LOVE

Wooden kitchen cupboard doors have a tendency to become sticky and then look unsightly and feel nasty. Stop this happening by regularly wiping them down with a cloth soaked in a warm solution of washing-up liquid with a capful of vinegar – take care not to overwet the wood, though. Rinse with another clean cloth wrung out with plain water, then buff dry.

•••

BACK TO THE CHOPPING BOARD

A chopping board can become notoriously smelly, particularly if you like cooking with onions and garlic. To freshen it up, rub the surface with any type of vinegar mixed with a little mustard powder, leave overnight, then scrub under a hot tap, rinse, and leave it to dry on its side.

•••

TOP BRASS

Vinegar and salt work very well on brass that's badly in need of cleaning. Pour any type of vinegar onto a damp cloth, sprinkle with salt and get rubbing the tarnished brass (tip: if you have any cuts to your fingers, wear rubber gloves). The metal will instantly take on a lovely shine. Rinse under the tap and buff dry with a soft cotton cloth to finish.

BATHROOM

SHOWER WITH COMPLIMENTS

Take a look at your shower screen, which was once clear and sparkling. Is it now opaque and covered with drip marks, soap scum and grotty bits of limescale? Bring it back to its pristine past: mix some bicarbonate of soda and clear vinegar to a smooth paste and then, using a nylon scourer, apply a layer of the mixture to the shower screen (as well as to any ceramic tiles); you'll need to exercise a little elbow grease, too, which won't do any harm to the screen. Leave for a few minutes then rinse off and buff dry to a gleaming shine using a microfibre cloth for glass/mirrors (the smooth, slinky type that's similar to what you have in your glasses case for specs-cleaning) or, if you don't have one of those, a few sheets of scrunched-up kitchen paper will do just as well.

•••

BRILLIANT BATH AND BASIN

Here's a very effective, mildly abrasive but definitely non-scratchy cleaner for your bath and washbasins. In a bowl, mix together a loose paste of washing-up liquid, bicarbonate of soda and clear vinegar. Apply the mixture to the surface with a damp cloth, rubbing gently to clean away the dirt, then rinse down.

• • •

PUT THE SPARKLE BACK INTO YOUR SHOWERHEAD

Is your chrome showerhead caked with limescale and the water flow really poor? Unscrew it and steep it overnight in a bowl filled with equal quantities of clear vinegar and water. By morning the scale will have miraculously softened and can be peeled off easily. Use a nylon scourer to remove any last stubborn bits. Note: don't use this on special metal finishes, as the acid in the vinegar can easily damage the surface.

• • •

TAKE THE GROT OUT OF YOUR GROUT

Grouting lines between tiles are absorbent and so latch onto scum and mildew – not a great look! Scrub these areas clean with a damp toothbrush dipped in a paste made of bicarbonate of soda with a few drops of vinegar and bleach, then rinse and buff dry.

• • •

KEEP LIMESCALE IN THE LOO AT BAY

It's one thing having limescale in your loo, but when it turns brown it's a step too far. Salts and iron in water cause this, so you need to treat the limescale itself. One good way is to dissolve 250g citric acid powder (available from the chemist or a DIY shop) in a 5-litre bucket of hot water and pour slowly into the bowl. It'll start to fizz as it dissolves the limescale, so swish it around with a loo brush to help. When the fizzing stops, flush. Repeat if necessary. Keep the scale at bay by pouring a bottle of clear vinegar into the bowl about once a month; leave overnight before flushing away.

• • •

DECLOG THE BATH WASTE

Are you a fan of bath oil? If so, you could be in danger of clogging up the plughole as the oil attracts and collects hair, which eventually bungs up pipes and drains. If you notice that your bath is emptying more slowly than usual, pour a cup each of washing soda crystals and salt down the plughole, then add a cup of clear vinegar followed by a kettle of boiling water. Simultaneously have a go with the plunger – you might be horrified at what could emerge… but far better out than in. Rubber gloves are always a good idea if you're a bit squeamish.

• • •

A WEE PROBLEM SOLVED

As the mum of two males, I know that if you have small (or even big) boys living with you, you can be sure that some pee will land on the wall behind the cistern, leading to nasty niffs. To zap it immediately, wash with a 50:50 solution of vinegar and warm water. In the long run, it's best to ensure boys are aiming properly (why can't they just sit on the loo like the rest of us?). Supervise your small men, and make sure they press *down* every time… and actually look at what they're doing! Also, get them into the habit of wiping the rim of the pan afterwards – it'll soon become automatic.

LAUNDRY

SWEET-SMELLING BABY CLOTHES

Do you have a baby or small child at home? Add a cup of clear vinegar to each washload of baby clothes during the rinse cycle. This will break down the uric acid and leave the clothes lovely and soft as well as smelling fresh.

• • •

KEEP YOUR POWDER DRY

If your washing machine isn't taking all the powder from the detergent drawer, check you're storing it properly – the powder will be sticky or hard if it's in a damp place. If the detergent isn't damp, it may be that the drawer's water jets are blocked. A water softener such as Calgon will help protect the heating element and other parts of your washing machine, but it won't stop limescale forming on the jets if you live in a hard-water area. To clean the jets, mix equal parts clear vinegar and water. Remove the drawer, then scrub the solution onto the roof of the empty compartment. Now run an idle wash – have the drum empty, set the machine to the hottest programme and add the maximum dose of detergent.

SOFT TOWELS GUARANTEED

Overusing fabric conditioner will actually make towels less absorbent and hard. If there's a build-up it never actually gets rinsed out, and every time you use the washing machine, more and more is added and gets left behind. This will eventually make coloured fabrics look dull and whites grey. To keep the fluff factor in your towels, check you're using enough detergent and include softener only every second or third time you wash them. Other times, use the same amount of clear vinegar as you would conditioner – add half a cup to the first rinse (tip it into the detergent drawer while the machine is filling with water). This is how they launder them commercially, which is probably why hotel towels stay so fluffy (and no – they won't smell vinegary). Finally, rinse and spin well (this way you'll eject more hard-water impurities). Line-drying helps to keep fibres fluffy; radiators do the opposite.

• • •

IT'S THE PITS

How annoying is it when the armpits of your favourite shirts turn yellow and hard from sweat, and after a while normal washing just won't hack it? Soak the stained area overnight in a solution of half clear vinegar, half water, then machine-wash as normal.

• • •

BACK TO BLACK

When a black item turns an unappealing shade of grey over a number of washes, chances are this is because of a build-up of detergent left in the fabric, rather than actual loss of black dye. To sort this, soak the item for a few hours in a sink filled with warm water with a little clear vinegar. Afterwards, rinse thoroughly and machine-wash as normal.

• • •

SMOKE GETS UP YOUR NOSE

Admittedly this is not an everyday occurrence, but house fires do happen. If you're in the unfortunate position of trying to rescue smoke-damaged clothes, bedlinen and towels that are stinking, first sprinkle everything with bicarbonate of soda, then machine-wash twice, adding a cupful of vinegar to the drum for each cycle. If possible, hang everything outside on a washing line (which will help to get rid of the smell).

• • •

SEAL WITH A SPRITZ

Nasty germs and smelly mould can lurk in your washing-machine seal. Mix equal quantities of water and clear vinegar in a spray bottle and squirt onto the inside of the seal. Leave for a few minutes then wipe clean.

• • •

LOOK AFTER YOUR IRON AND IT WILL LOOK AFTER YOU

Most steam irons nowadays have some type of self-cleaning or anti-calc system – use these once a month according to the instructions on the packet and from the manufacturer. If your iron doesn't have this feature, pour equal parts clear vinegar and tap water into the reservoir until it's about one-third full. Turn the heat to medium and allow the iron to steam for 5–10 minutes until all the vinegar evaporates. Switch off the iron, then fill the reservoir with fresh water. Turn on the iron again to flush through any leftover mineral deposits and vinegar. Switch off, allow to cool, then wipe the base with a soft clean cloth. If you think the steam vents are still clogged, clear with a cotton bud dipped in water with a little vinegar added. To help stop any future build-up of limescale, pour away excess water when you've finished ironing.

LIVING ROOM

WOOD YOU BELIEVE IT?

Spray furniture polish is all well and good for a quick fix (and makes the place smell as if it's been newly spring-cleaned), but in the long term layers of silicon in the polish can build up on wooden furniture and leave the surfaces annoyingly tacky. Instead, here's a lovely natural treatment that won't leave you with sticky surfaces. Mix together two-parts olive oil to one-part white wine vinegar and apply the tiniest amount to a soft cotton cloth. Apply a thin layer to the wood, leave for a few minutes, then buff to a sheen with another soft clean cloth. Solid-wood furniture needs a polish only about twice a year; use a teeny amount of wax and buff well to get a good shine. Dust regularly and treat any occasional sticky marks with a chamois leather wrung out in a solution of one-part clear vinegar to six-parts water.

• • •

BEAUTY SPOTS SORTED

How often has your mascara or lipstick mysteriously leapt from your hand and landed on the (beige or cream) carpet? Speed is important here. Mix one-part clear vinegar to two-parts warm water and dab, dab, dab (don't rub, as you might damage the pile) with a clean white cotton cloth.

• • •

IT'S CURTAINS FOR MOULD

During cold weather, with radiators at full blast and not much ventilation going through the house, this is the time of year you might notice spots of mildew on your curtain linings. If they're dry clean only, the cleaner will deal with the spores but probably not manage the stains. However, what you can try at home is to gather them up and take them outside (so the unhealthy spores don't spread around the room), wipe them down with a solution of warm water and detergent, then rinse with a cloth wrung out in clear vinegar. The less time the mould has had to form, the easier it'll be to zap the stains.

• • •

SMOKE OUT THOSE STAINS

To remove smoke marks from brickwork around a fireplace, first clean the whole surface with a soft brush or the upholstery tool of the vacuum cleaner. Now dip a scrubbing brush into a bucket of warm water plus a cup of clear vinegar and go at the bricks with the brush. Rinse off afterwards.

• • •

SOFA SO GOOD

Had a beer spillage on the sofa and it's left a stain after you thought you'd cleaned it? Make up a solution of one-part vinegar to five-parts warm water and sponge carefully but thoroughly (test for colourfastness on a small area on the back of the sofa), then go over it with a cotton cloth and clear warm water. Leave it to dry naturally.

•••

SAY GOODBYE TO THE BIG SMOKE

Have you bought or been given furniture that belonged to a smoker? If you yourself don't smoke, once you get it home it'll smell strongly of stale tobacco. Here's what to do: wipe down the whole thing, whatever it is, with clear vinegar, then leave to dry overnight. Next day, coat in a light dusting of bicarbonate of soda and leave for a few hours before wiping off, again with a cloth that has been wrung out in vinegar.

•••

IT'S A DOG'S LIFE

If your doggie has had a naughty wee on your living-room carpet, you can get rid of the smell with a solution of three-parts soda water and one-part clear vinegar. Also, by using vinegar the dog won't now recognise the smell as 'theirs' and will go elsewhere to do their business (hopefully outside rather than to a different room).

OTHER
INGENIOUS USES

NOT A TRACE LEFT

You know that annoying white tidemark that appears on your lovely leather boots after you've been out in the snow? And how it keeps on reappearing, even after you've polished them? Here's the answer: rub a little vinegar on cotton wool over the white marks before repolishing. All traces will be gone and they'll look like new again.

•••

EXHAUST THOSE FUMES

You're decorating indoors, the room is filling up with strong paint fumes and your head starts thumping… it's time to cut through and neutralise the effects of the strong smells by placing an open dish of vinegar in the room.

•••

39

GREASE IS THE WORD

If you enjoy waxing your car but hate it when wax lands on the windscreen or windows (normally so difficult to shift!), give the glass a wipe with good old neat vinegar. Rinse off then buff dry with a microfibre cloth for glass and mirrors.

• • •

HAVE A MELTDOWN

Why is it that the very morning the car is all frosted up, there's no de-icer spray or scraper to be found anywhere? And that credit-card trick takes for-flaming-ever. A good remedy is to mix three-parts warm water to one-part clear vinegar in a spray bottle and go for it. (This mix is great for cleaning the glass at the same time.)

• • •

FOR QUICK CLEAN-UPS

Once your washing-up liquid bottle is empty, instead of throwing it away, fill it with clear vinegar (don't forget to label it) for quick clean-ups. It's great for shower doors and it's lighter and safer than lugging around a vinegar bottle made of glass.

• • •

HAIR TODAY, GONE TOMORROW

If you're a fan of hairspray, you might notice a rough residue forming over hard surfaces, which can be tricky to shift. Wiping over with clear vinegar will remove it in an instant.

• • •

CHEW ON THIS

You wear dentures and you've run out of cleaning tablets. Here's the answer: leave them in a solution of half clear vinegar and half warm water for around 15 minutes, then brush well under a running tap.

...

FOR A CLEAR CHEST

Is there a Victorian pine chest that doesn't stink of mothballs? The smell will gradually fade over time, but meanwhile you can air the chest by leaving the drawers open and washing all the surfaces and drawers with a damp cloth and warm soapy water (be careful not to over-wet any areas) mixed with a cupful of clear vinegar. Leave in a warm room to dry quickly, then place some tumble-drier sheets in the empty drawers and keep them closed for about a month.

...

STRICTLY FOR THE BIRDS

A birdbath is a lovely thing to have in the garden, but when it's covered in slime and algae, less so. Bale out any water and, with equal parts vinegar and water and using an old toothbrush, give the bath a good scrub and hose it down with fresh water before refilling. The birds will love you for it.

...

DON'T BE WEEDY

If you have annoying weeds in paving cracks – which, if you tackled them individually would take forever to pull out, plus do in your back – crush them all in one swoop with vinegar diluted 50:50 with hot water. Pour this into a small watering can or spray bottle and douse the lot. After a few hours they'll shrivel up and die off.

• • •

SHINY SHOES

Fancy seeing your reflection in your patent leather shoes or handbag? Moisten a soft cotton cloth with a little clear vinegar and wipe over the leather.

• • •

GET OUT OF A SCRAPE

A friend was recently stripping wallpaper, which seemed to be taking forever – particularly the last bits, when energy and enthusiasm were in very limited supply. Then she had a eureka moment: she added a cup of vinegar to her bucket of warm water, washed over the residue with it… and all of a sudden the scraping became a lot easier.

• • •

THE SOFT APPROACH

You've done that thing of not cleaning paintbrushes properly at the end of decorating, and next time you go to your brush, it's rock hard. Don't throw it away until you try this fix. Bring 300ml of any type of vinegar to the boil, pour it into a clean jam-jar then plunge in the brush. Leave for a few hours then wash out the bristles in warm soapy water.

• • •

I CAN SEE CLEARLY NOW...

Clean dirty prescription glasses or sunglasses with a 1:1 solution of water and clear vinegar. Just rub it over the lenses and rinse off. Leave to dry naturally. Resist using shirt tails or a t-shirt to dry the lenses, as they often contain lots of bacteria or fibres that'll scratch the glass.

• • •

A CANNY WAY TO CATCH PESKY FRUIT FLIES

It takes just a small spot of rotting fruit for a cloud of fruit flies to gather and are a particular pest in the summer when fruit ripens far too quickly. Mould spots can appear overnight from seemingly perfect fruit, such as peaches and figs. To catch those little bugs, pour a dash of vinegar into a ramekin, add a dot of washing-up liquid then cover with clingfilm. Push holes in the clingfilm all over the top and put near the offending fruit bowl. The next day they'll have dived into the pool and be floating in the liquid.

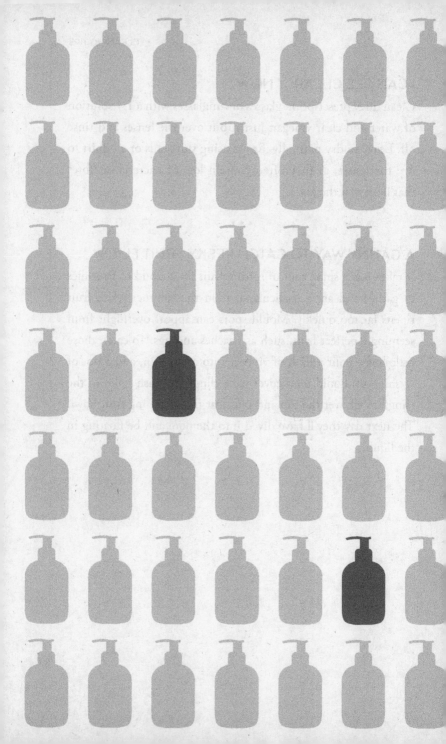

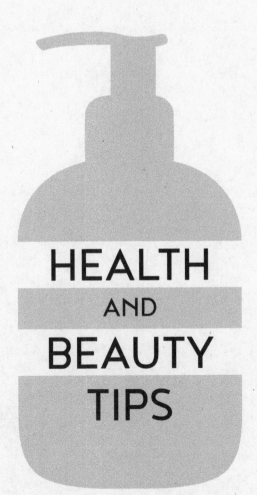

HEALTH
AND
BEAUTY
TIPS

Move over, kale smoothie – cider vinegar seems to have stolen your place. And it's believed to be not only beneficial for the digestive and immune systems but also for skin complaints and fungal infections.

Including diluted organic cider vinegar daily and sparingly in your diet, particularly before mealtimes, could have a beneficial effect on your cholesterol levels. But sparingly is key: drinking more than a few tablespoons a day is not advisable as it could cause stomach cramps and, in extreme cases, erode the stomach lining. Japanese rice vinegars are gaining ground too and thought to help prevent inflammation and hypertension.

Cider vinegar's reputation was boosted early in 2018 when Victoria Beckham encouraged her Instagram followers to take two tablespoons on rising, on an empty tum. Other celebrity cider vinegar fans include Katy Perry, Jennifer Aniston and Scarlett Johansson, who apparently uses it on her face to keep her complexion clear. With manufacturers claiming other benefits such as reducing the risk of heart disease and helping weight loss, sales of Ocado's 5-litre cider vinegar bottles went up by 43% that year.

Of course, retailers have cottoned onto this trend and now you'll find an array of vinegar-based soft drinks on the supermarket shelves, often fizzy and sweetened, marketed as health-boosting and detoxifying grown-up concoctions. Time will tell how beneficial they are, but they're bound to be better for you than a can of cola...

SILKY SKIN
SOLUTIONS

SCRUB FOR GARDENERS

Here's a quick-to-mix scrub that will clean dirty hands after a weekend spent in the garden weeding and pruning. Put 5 tablespoons of coarse sea salt into a bowl, add 1 tablespoon of cider vinegar, a few dashes of lavender oil and 1 teaspoon of olive oil and mix together, then pour into a jam-jar – this makes enough for a small jar. To use, spoon it into the palm of your hands and rub well, paying particular attention to any ingrained dirt. Rinse well, then dry your hands. As well as being a great cleanser, it also leaves your skin beautifully moisturised and scented.

•••

TONE GREASY SKIN

Soothe an outbreak of spots or greasy skin with this DIY toner that you can quickly make up as and when you need to use it. Put 2 tablespoons of cool boiled water into a ramekin with 1 teaspoon of cider vinegar and 2 teaspoons of rosewater. Stir together and use a cotton pad to sweep it over your face after cleansing.

• • •

KNOCK SPOTS OFF BAD SKIN
Acne and skin boils can be treated with cider vinegar, which should reduce both pain and inflammation. Dab a little onto the affected area with a cotton wool pad – it may well sting but that's a sign that the antiseptic elements are active in fighting the bacteria.

• • •

SUFFERING FROM DRY SKIN?
When moisture is sapped from your skin through central heating or a hot holiday and no amount of moisturiser will soothe those parts, run a warm (not hot) bath and pour in around 200ml distilled vinegar. Swirl it around to disperse then step in and enjoy. Throw in a big handful of Epsom salts to relieve aching muscles at the same time, if you like.

• • •

SOOTHE YOUR SUNBURN
If you've overdone it in the sun, soak a flannel with distilled malt vinegar (the clear kind) and gently dab it onto the affected areas. This is particularly effective if the vinegar's been chilled. The vinegar will help prevent itchiness, reduce blistering and subsequent skin peeling.

TREATMENTS FOR HEALTHY-LOOKING HAIR

FANCY GOING 'POO-FREE'?

This sounds weird, but this is the phrase given to those who give up washing their hair with shampoo and other haircare products – not what you might be thinking! The idea is that the longer you go without using shampoo, the better the natural oils in hair can build up and condition your hair. Washing your hair just in warm water as you shower or bathe will refresh it while you get used to the feeling of not using shampoo, but if you want to condition it, give it a vinegar rinse once a week. Fill a cup with warm water and add 2 tablespoons of cider vinegar. Pour this over your hair then comb it through to get rid of any knots or tangles. Leave this on for around 3 minutes to allow it to work. You can give your scalp a good massage with your fingertips at the same time, which helps to increase circulation. Rinse well and dry as you normally do.

• • •

DOWN WITH DANDRUFF

Lose those tell-tale scalp flakes on your shoulders with this store-cupboard remedy. Before shampooing, mix 4 tablespoons of cider vinegar (it's naturally anti-fungal) and 4 tablespoons of water in a bowl. Pour over dry hair and massage in, then shampoo as normal. Continue to use this once a week until the dandruff clears.

• • •

NIP NITS IN THE BUD

Vinegar won't kill head lice but it will help deal with the eggs (nits) stuck to your hair, which will stop new lice from hatching. Using a medicated shampoo before you do the vinegar treatment will help ensure that the adult lice are dead, which will reduce the chances of the lice spreading.

Use clear vinegar – it's strong enough to dissolve the coatings on nits, but not acidic enough to irritate most people's skin. This needs to be done by someone other than the victim!

First dampen the hair with a little water, then pour on a few cups of neat vinegar. Massage this into the scalp and cover as much of the hair as possible, then leave on the hair for 5–10 minutes. Now run a nit comb (from a chemist) thoroughly through the hair – the loosened nits and some adult lice will be more easily removed. Examine the hair carefully for any remainers. When you think you've got all of the nits, rinse off the rest of the vinegar and towel-dry the hair. Make sure that particular towel is used only by the infected person until the head is completely clear.

PAMPER FEET
AND HANDS

FRESHEN STINKY FEET

Sometimes no amount of swooshing in the shower will rinse away pongy aromas. For a refreshing – if vinegary – foot bath, fill a washing-up bowl with 2 litres of warm water then pour in 200ml distilled vinegar, a couple of dashes of peppermint oil and 2 tablespoons of Epsom salts or magnesium flakes. Immerse your feet in the water and soak for 15 minutes. Dry well. Spritz with rosewater to freshen.

• • •

SOFTEN CUTICLES

Pushing your cuticles back extends the nail, but if you find they're tough and hard, soak them in vinegar first. Pour enough into a small bowl to dip your fingers into up to the first joint and add a couple of splashes of lavender oil. Pop in your fingertips and hold there for about 5 minutes. Rinse with warm water and dry well.

TIPS AND TRICKS FOR MAKE-UP ACCESSORIES

FRESHEN UP BEAUTY BRUSHES

Make-up brushes should be cleaned once a week to wash away bacteria and excess make-up. Pour enough warm boiled water into a small bowl to just cover the head of the brush and stir in 1 tablespoon of distilled white vinegar. Swirl the brush heads around in the water to release the dirt then rinse under the tap with warm water. Shake to remove excess water then leave to dry naturally.

• • •

GLOOPY NAIL VARNISH?

If your nail varnish has been hanging around for a while and seems too thick to brush on, soak a cotton pad in a little cider vinegar and wipe it over the nails. Pull the varnish brush out of the bottle, wiping half of it off as you go, then use as usual. The acid in the vinegar helps to thin the nail varnish, making it easier to paint on.

SOOTHING COLD TREATMENTS

SETTLE A SORE THROAT

Neat vinegar is a bit harsh to stomach, so instead try adding a tablespoon each of cider vinegar and honey to a cup of hot water. Sip this to help ease your symptoms; this is particularly effective if your sore throat is due to a bacterial infection, as it's thought that cider vinegar's anti-bacterial properties fight off the germs.

• • •

CLEAR NASAL CONGESTION

Fill a bowl with boiling water and add 3 tablespoons of cider vinegar. Then pop your head over the bowl and cover it with a towel to keep the steam in, close your eyes and inhale the vapour for a few minutes. This is effective because cider vinegar has high pH levels that break up phlegm and clear the throat. Repeat twice daily until the phlegm is gone.

EASE ACHES AND PAINS

CUT THE CRAMP

The combination of honey and vinegar is good for your circulation, which can help if you suffer from night-time leg cramps. Before bed, dissolve 2 tablespoons of cider vinegar and 1 tablespoon of honey in boiling water. If your cramp is more likely to happen while you're at the gym, take this before working out.

• • •

AID ACHING MUSCLES

When you exercise, your body uses oxygen to break down glucose for energy, and during intense exercise there may not be enough oxygen available to do this, in which case lactic acid is produced, which your body can convert into energy without oxygen. If lactic acid builds up, though, it can cause pain in the muscles. Cider vinegar helps to draw out lactic acid, so mix a few tablespoons of it into a cup of warm water, wet a flannel with this and plaster it onto any sore area for around 20 minutes for a soothing effect.

JOINT TREATMENT FOR ARTHRITIS

Some people swear by honey and vinegar (2 tablespoons each of honey and cider vinegar in a mug of warm water) to ease the symptoms of arthritis. This remedy can be bought ready mixed; for example, Honegar, which is available at Holland and Barrett. As a sufferer myself, I gave it a go, and I have been taking it ever since and continue to enjoy the benefits of it. I can't be sure, but I wonder if my symptoms would have worsened without it.

• • •

TAKE THE STING OUT OF AN INSECT BITE

Mix cider vinegar and cornflour into a thick paste and apply this directly to the affected area to take the edge off the pain.

• • •

OUT WITH GOUT

Soak the sore foot (or feet) for half an hour in a basin filled with hot water and cider vinegar at a ratio of 4:1. Alternatively, soak a clean, dry cloth in neat cider vinegar, wrap it around the affected area and leave for the same length of time.

• • •

CRUISING FOR A BRUISING?

Some people swear you can tone down both the swelling and colour of a bruise if you soak a cloth or a couple of sheets of kitchen paper in clear vinegar and apply them as soon as possible after the injury.

NASTY INFECTIONS

ALLEVIATE ATHLETE'S FOOT

This fungal infection can be a misery; it can lead to cracks and peeling skin between the toes and cause severe itchiness and pain. Fungal creams are generally prescribed, but not everyone can use them (some anti-fungals trigger an allergic reaction). An alternative is to bathe your tootsies each evening, using one-part clear vinegar to two-parts warm water. Dry between the toes carefully after use – dabbing rather than rubbing – and use a separate towel specifically for your feet. Wear clean cotton socks each day and ring the changes with shoes and boots. If athlete's foot is left untreated it can spread to your toenails and lead to unsightly (though painless) toenail fungus.

•••

FIGHT FUNGAL TOENAILS

A fungus thrives in an alkaline environment and loves dark, moist areas such as inside a shoe – ideal conditions for an infection to grow and spread to other toenails. Organic acidic cider vinegar (make sure it's the type that includes the mother – check the label) has natural antifungal properties that help prevent the fungus growing or spreading. It can also help restore the pH level of the nail and skin.

First cut back your toenails to the toe line, then, once a day, add two or three cups of cider vinegar, plus the same amount of warm water, to a basin. Make sure all the (cleaned) toes are submerged and sit for 20 minutes. Dry your feet thoroughly afterwards. Keep going with this treatment (use a fresh solution each time) until the infected nails grow out. Biona organic cider vinegar is available online in 5-litre containers.

HEALTHY FROM INSIDE OUT

THE ANSWER TO A BURNING QUESTION

If you're finding that acidic foods such as red wine vinegar trigger acid reflux and cause heartburn, it's worth trying a posher, aged red wine vinegar. The lengthened production time gives a smoother, less sharp taste – yes, it's still sour but it is perhaps gentler on your system (see page 15).

• • •

A SWELL SOLUTION

Cider vinegar contains potassium, which helps prevent water retention. When potassium levels in the body are low, cells start to fill with water, which causes swelling in various parts of the body (the ankles are an obvious area). Treat swollen ankles by soaking a small towel in a 4:1 solution of warm water and cider vinegar, then wrap them in it for 10 minutes. Repeat this process with cold water to further reduce swelling.

• • •

ALLEVIATE MORNING SICKNESS

If you're feeling queasy during your pregnancy, as soon as you rise, drink a glass of hot water with a teaspoon of cider vinegar added.

• • •

LOOSEN THINGS UP

Cider vinegar, like other fermented foods such as yogurt and sauerkraut, contains healthy bacteria that populate your gut and help digestion. Cider vinegar also contains pectin, a water-soluble fibre that can help improve your overall through-put. Take 1 tablespoon with the same amount of honey in a glass of hot water each morning.

GIVE YOUR BODY A BOOST

BLACK MAGIC

Black vinegar – also known as brown rice vinegar – is made from fermented unpolished rice and malt and is used as a tonic in Chinese and Japanese cultures. It contains amino acids, vitamins, minerals and other nutrients. It's thought that the high levels of antioxidants it contains may have the potential to prevent or even heal the damage caused to the body's cells by free radical activity, and consequently may help prevent some types of cancer. Take 1 tablespoon with the same amount of honey in a cup of hot water each morning.

• • •

SLIM PICKINGS

Our bodies need amino acids to build muscle; the more muscle strength you have, the better able your body is to use up calories, even when resting. The citric acid in black vinegar is a natural blocker of starch, which helps regulate your blood sugar and lessen the absorption of fat. This is another good reason to take

1 tablespoon of vinegar with the same amount of honey in a cup of hot water each morning.

• • •

BOOST YOUR IMMUNE SYSTEM

Rice vinegar contains essential amino acids, which help to boost immunity and are known to fight the development of lactic acid in the blood (which leads to stiffness and tiredness, see Aid Aching Muscles, page 56). Holding down lactic acid levels helps to keep up your energy levels during the day. Incorporate rice vinegar into your cooking and salad dressings.

• • •

MAKE FRIENDS WITH ANTIOXIDANTS

These are present in the grapes used to produce red wine (and also red wine vinegar) and are thought to protect the body from damage to cells that occurs when it is exposed to environmental poisons such as exhaust fumes and cigarette smoke. Olives are also a good source of antioxidants, so it's a good-health idea to make your vinaigrette with olive oil and red wine vinegar rather than lemon juice.

AND THAT'S NOT ALL...

TIME TO RELAX

If you have a headache due to stress or tension, lightly dampen a cloth with white wine vinegar infused with a few drops of rosemary oil, put it across your forehead, lie down in a quiet room with some soothing music, close your eyes and relax.

•••

BLAST THAT COLD SORE

If you've ever had one of these, you'll know that they can be very painful, unsightly and annoyingly slow to heal. If you're susceptible, as soon as you feel that warning tingle, dab some cider vinegar directly onto the area. If you've ignored the tingle and the sore is established, mix a teaspoon of lemon juice with the same amount of vinegar and apply directly to the sore.

•••

HELP FOR HICCUPS

Next time you or someone in your family gets a bout of uncontrollable hiccups, try drinking a teaspoon of neat cider vinegar. It's unclear how or why this might work, but one theory is that it's the shock of the acidity that brings the spasms to a stop. Worth a try!

• • •

NO FLEAS PLEASE

Mix half vinegar (any kind) and half water in a spray bottle and spritz your cat's fur once a day.

RECIPES

RECIPES

Vinegar is having something of a renaissance right now and is being used in so many more ways than adding a touch of acidity to dressings and dips. From marinades and stews to baking and desserts, this store-cupboard staple can play a part in any recipe you're cooking, whatever time of day.

It's no longer the preserve of our Friday night fish-and-chip feast, where malt vinegar is splashed liberally over hot-from-the-fryer chips along with a dusting of fine salt. It's being used in lots of restaurants to 'finish' dishes – whether the call is to add oomph to a pan sauce that tastes bland or a drizzle to accentuate ingredients on a just-plated salad.

This interest is also reflected in supermarket sales (different stores have reported anything from 50-60% increases in 2018). Glance along any supermarket shelf and, stacked neatly alongside the oils, there are plenty of brands to pick and choose from. Malt has been moved aside to make room for red and white wine vinegar and its single grape varieties and there's also a choice of traditional brown balsamic and a lighter-tasting white. In independent delis, online shops and specialist food stores, you'll probably find an even wider selection including flavoured vinegars. Read on for more easy tips and tricks on how to use them...

QUICK AND
LIGHT MEALS

Pressed for time and need to grab a bite to eat? Take inspiration from these recipes achievable in minutes. Scoot through the vegetable drawer for leftover treasures and gather all those bits and pieces to make a sumptuous soup. Lightened with a splash of vinegar, it softens the sweetness for a distinct savoury touch. There's also the best way to poach eggs – yes, vinegar's essential – plus a recipe for a twist on Turkish eggs and other glorious treats.

USE VINEGAR TO POACH EGGS

Adding a tablespoon of vinegar to bubbling water when you are poaching eggs helps to coagulate the white and stop it spreading in the water. For the best results, choose a wide pan and half-fill it with water. Cover and bring to a good bubble. Turn down the heat a little so the water is just simmering and pour in the vinegar. Crack each egg into a cup and slowly lower it into the water, dropping each egg into a different space. Cook the eggs for 3 minutes. Line a plate with kitchen paper, then lift out with a slotted spoon and drain on the kitchen paper to soak up excess water before serving.

ENJOY IN THIS UNUSUAL COMBINATION...

Poached eggs sitting on a bed of creamy natural yogurt and drizzled in oil is called *çilbir* in Turkey, or Turkish eggs. The yogurt is seasoned with crushed garlic and the oil, often mixed with the spice Aleppo pepper, turns it into a very savoury affair. Here's a twist, perfect for any time of day.

Serves 4

300g Greek yogurt
4 free-range eggs
4 ripe tomatoes
1 tbsp extra virgin olive oil
1 tsp red wine vinegar
Small handful dill, chopped
Pinch of chilli flakes
Sea salt

1 Spoon the yogurt into a bowl, season with a pinch of salt and beat in 2 tablespoons of cold water. Divide between four bowls and smooth out into a round nest, leaving a little dip in the middle.

2 Poach the eggs, following the instructions above. Meanwhile, chop the tomatoes and put them in a bowl with the olive oil, red wine vinegar, dill and chilli flakes before stirring everything together.

3 When the eggs are cooked, drain, then spoon into the middle of each bowl on top of the yogurt. Dress each with the tomato salad and serve.

RICH PICKINGS FROM THE VEGETABLE DRAWER

Here's a sweep-through-the-vegetable-drawer pasta dish that's sharpened with a splash of balsamic vinegar. The sauce is paired with orzo pasta – those little rice-like shapes also used in soups – which makes the finished dish resemble a veg-rich risotto. The balsamic vinegar only feels like a dash at the end, but it brings all the flavours sharply into focus by providing that perfect touch of acidity.

Serves 2

3 tbsp olive oil
½ red or white onion, finely sliced
2 garlic cloves, sliced
1–2 carrots, diced
½ red pepper, deseeded and diced
1 small courgette, diced
Small handful of cavolo nero or kale, finely chopped
Large handful of shelled peas
100g orzo pasta
6 baby plum tomatoes, quartered
1 tbsp balsamic vinegar
Small handful of chopped parsley and basil
Sea salt and freshly ground black pepper

1 Heat the olive oil in a medium pan, then add the onion and garlic. Season and cook for around 5 minutes. Add the carrots, pepper and courgette to the pan and stir everything together. Toss in the cavolo nero or kale, then throw in the peas. Cook for about 10 minutes over the lowest heat until the garlic has started to turn golden and the vegetables have softened.

2 Meanwhile, bring a medium pan of salted water to the boil. Add the orzo pasta to the water and cook for 7–10 minutes until tender.

3 Stir 1 tablespoon of the pasta cooking water into the vegetables, along with the baby plum tomatoes, balsamic vinegar, chopped parsley and basil. Drain the orzo, then stir in to the vegetables, season to taste and heat for a minute or two before dividing between two bowls.

SPICED CHICKPEAS FOR FISH, CHICKEN, SALAD, YOGURT OR HUMMUS

You can pick up these ubiquitous pulses for less than a pound, even in a corner shop, and they really do offer value for money. The chickpeas themselves, of course, can be tipped into soups and stews, salads or whizzed with olive oil, garlic and cumin to make hummus. The drained liquid is valuable, too. Known as aquafaba (water of beans), it's a dead-ringer for egg whites in vegan recipes, and in the same way, it needs to be whipped first until it's looking thick, white and glossy before being used in either meringues or mousse (see page 146).

This recipe is uber-versatile and really does fit any occasion... The warm dressing of olive oil, garlic, spice and chilli livens up a drained can or carton of chickpeas and is flavoursome enough to serve as a side with a roast, a piece of fish or meat, or a few slices of griddled tofu. Don't let the vinegar cook for very long at all in this dressing – you need that sharpness to add contrast to the overall flavour.

For a starter or quick lunch, spoon a small tub of hummus into a large flat bowl and spread out with the back of a spoon so it looks like a pool. Spoon the chickpeas over the top and snip over some herbs if you have them.

Serves 4

2 tbsp extra virgin olive oil
1 garlic clove, sliced
½ tsp cumin seeds
½ mild red chilli, deseeded and chopped
400g can chickpeas, drained
1 tbsp cider vinegar

1   Heat the oil in a frying pan over a medium heat. Stir in the garlic and cumin seeds and cook for about 30 seconds until the garlic just starts to turn golden. Add the chilli and chickpeas, season well, and continue to cook for a minute or two to heat everything through. Pour in the vinegar, stir again and serve.

HOT SMOKY CHICKEN FOR A BUN

Slicing chicken breast across the grain cuts it into thin pieces, ideal for cooking quickly in a hot pan. Tossing them first in a marinade of red wine vinegar, herbs and spices ensures they're really tender with lots of flavour. You can do this up to two days ahead, too – just store in a sealable container in the fridge. Serve in a bun with mayonnaise, lettuce, sliced onion and tomatoes.

Serves 2

1 tbsp red wine vinegar
1 tsp freshly chopped thyme or rosemary
2 garlic cloves, sliced
½ tsp smoked paprika
2 large, skinless, boneless chicken breasts (around 400g)
1 tbsp olive oil
Sea salt and freshly ground black pepper

1   Start by mixing the marinade in a container, which helps the spice to dissolve into the vinegar first. This makes it much easier to coat the chicken evenly. Put the vinegar into the container with the chopped thyme or rosemary, garlic and smoked paprika and season well.

2   Next, lay the chicken breasts on a board and use a sharp knife to cut each into pieces horizontally. You should be able to cut around five slices from each one. Drop into the vinegar mixture and toss around to ensure they are coated. Drizzle over the olive oil and toss again.

3   Heat a large frying pan until hot. Turn the heat down to medium then cook the chicken in batches for 2–3 minutes on each side. To make sure they're cooked, split one of the thick pieces open – there should be no pink bits inside. Set aside to rest for a minute or two before serving.

FOR AN ALTERNATIVE SIDE

Don't fancy a bun? Serve with steamed potatoes and green beans (French or runner), tossed in a knob of butter.

IF YOU PREFER MORE PUNCH

Add 2 thickly sliced garlic cloves to the marinade; when you start to cook the chicken, leave out the garlic until the end, as it can burn if you cook it for too long and taste bitter. Once all the chicken pieces have cooked, stir the slices into the hot pan with an extra drizzle of oil. Cook until just golden and spoon over the top.

ONE-PAN PEANUT BUTTER NOODLES

Here's a recipe that can be served in many different ways but is just as good on its own. Cooled and chilled, it also makes a budget-friendly take-to-work lunch. This quantity serves two but can be easily multiplied to feed more and can be zhuzhed up with a handful of frozen peas, some finely chopped (wilted, even) spring onions and strips of carrot. Or you can make it more of a feast by topping it with chopped tofu or a fried egg for vegetarians, or pan-fried prawns, shredded leftover chicken or pork for fish and meat lovers.

Serves 2

2 nests of medium egg noodles
2 tbsp peanut butter
1 tsp sesame oil
1 tbsp soy sauce
1 tbsp rice vinegar (or use white wine vinegar)
Sea salt and white pepper

1   Bring a medium pan of water to the boil and cook the egg noodles for 4 minutes until tender to the bite.

2   While the noodles are cooking, put the peanut butter into a bowl, add the sesame oil, soy sauce, vinegar and season with salt and white pepper.

3   When the noodles are cooked, add 1 tablespoon of cooking water to the dressing and whisk in. Drain the noodles well and return to the pan, along with the dressing. Swirl everything around in the heat of the pan until the noodles are coated.

4   Divide between two bowls and serve.

MAKE THE MOST OF WIZENED VEG

When you're rooting through the bottom of the vegetable drawer at the end of the week, resist the temptation to throw away those less-than-handsome bits and pieces lurking there. Try this side dish to liven them up. It's also a good way of finishing off that last scraping of cream cheese in an almost-empty tub.

Start by cooking the vegetables quickly until they're just tender, then, while the pan is still warm, use it to make a dressing from a little cooking water, some mustard and cream cheese and a splash of vinegar to cut through the creamy taste of the cheese.

Chop or shred around 500g vegetables into chunks and put into a medium pan. Pour over enough boiling water to cover, pop a lid on and bring to the boil. Simmer until just tender. Drain well, leaving a tablespoon or two of water in the pan at the end. Return the veg to the pan and put over a low heat. Add 1 teaspoon of red or white wine vinegar, 1 heaped teaspoon of wholegrain mustard and 1–2 tablespoons of cream cheese. Season and stir everything together. Great with steak, chicken, pork or even on toast if you've nothing else in.

MAINS

Don't save the vinegar for splashing on chips… here are ways to zhuzh up all sorts of ingredients and recipes. From slow-roasting a glut of plum tomatoes until soft and tender – with ideas to enjoy them in a simple supper – to adding it to a simmering meat stew to cut through the fat. It's also useful both as a marinade in a traditional and wonderfully rich pork vindaloo or a finishing touch when you've pan-fried a couple of bangers…

FRIDAY NIGHT STEAK AND SIDES - TWO WAYS

Rib-eye steak is the cut to choose for these recipes, the one where the fat is marbled all the way through the meat, which melts into the flesh as it cooks and gives it lots of flavour. One thick steak weighing around 300g will stretch to serve 2 and becomes even more of a bargain if you can find a butcher who does an offer, such as two for the price of one (usually on Fridays).

Once the steak is cooked, rest it for a couple of minutes to let the juices out, then drizzle these over at the end.

Both of these recipes take little more than 20 minutes to put together. The first dresses the steak in balsamic vinegar; the rich dark flavours provide a great contrast to the creamy, savoury blue cheese dressing, which is rustled up while the steak is cooking in the pan. Match with crisp chicory, cut into wedges.

The second uses vinegar and boiling water to tenderise and soften the flavour of slivered shallots first. They are then cooked in the pan juices with butter and vinegar for a toothsome sauce. It's so moreish, expect to find yourself wanting to lick the plate clean once everything else has gone…

BALSAMIC STEAK WITH ROQUEFORT DRESSING

Serves 2

1 tbsp olive oil
Sea salt and freshly ground black pepper
1 rib-eye steak, around 300g
2 tsp balsamic vinegar

For the dressing

30g Roquefort cheese
30g Greek yogurt
1 tbsp extra virgin olive oil
2 tsp red wine vinegar
1 red chicory bulb, halved
Handful of freshly chopped flat-leaf parsley

1   Heat all the oil in a frying pan over a medium heat. Season the steak well on each side then lay it down in the pan (you should hear a really good sizzle as it goes down). Cook for 4 minutes, lowering the heat if it looks as though the fat is spitting. Turn the steak over and cook for a further 4 minutes.

2   Meanwhile, put the Roquefort, yogurt, oil and vinegar into a small blender (or use a handheld one and a bowl). Season and add 1 teaspoon of cold water and whiz until smooth. When the steak has finished cooking, spoon over the balsamic vinegar. Lift onto a plate to rest for a few minutes.

3   Slice the steak into thin strips, divide between two plates and drizzle over the rested juices. Add the halved chicory, drizzle over the Roquefort sauce and scatter over the parsley.

RIB-EYE STEAK WITH BALSAMIC SHALLOTS

Serves 2

2 banana shallots, sliced lengthways into thin slivers
1 tbsp red wine vinegar
1 tsp olive oil
1 rib-eye steak (around 300g)
10g butter
1 tsp balsamic vinegar
Sea salt and freshly ground black pepper

1   Put the shallots into a bowl, add the vinegar and pour over enough boiling water to cover. Set aside.

2   Heat the oil in a pan over a medium heat and season the steak well. As soon as the oil is hot, lay the steak in the pan (again, it should really sizzle as it goes down) and cook for 4 minutes. Turn over and cook on the other side for 4 minutes. Lift out of the pan and set aside on a plate.

3   Put the butter in the same pan and as soon as it's melted, stir in the drained shallots. Season well and cook over a low heat for 5 minutes. Strain in the rested juices from the steak and stir in the balsamic vinegar and cook for 30 seconds.

4   Slice the steak and divide between two plates. Spoon over the shallots and serve with a crisp salad. Great with a cold beer.

QUICK NOTE...

This is the place to use up leftover soft herbs, as you only need a few to add a dash of colour and flavour to the shallots at the end. Parsley or chives are good, as is peppery rocket or watercress.

SPECIAL SLOW-ROASTED TOMATOES

Yes, you can roast tomatoes a quicker way – in the oven at a high temperature – but give them a little more time, at a much lower setting, and you'll be rewarded with these jewels.

A splash of vinegar is used here in the dressing and also added at the end, and it's this magical touch of acidity that really enhances the flavour of the tomatoes. A long, slow cook makes them taste far sweeter, too, with a moreish soft texture. You won't need many to make an impact. Store in a sealed container in the fridge for up to five days.

Serves 4-6

500g midi plum tomatoes on the vine, cut in half
2 tbsp extra virgin olive oil
1 tsp sherry vinegar, plus extra to serve
1 tsp each freshly chopped thyme and rosemary
Sea salt and freshly ground black pepper

1 Preheat the oven to 150°C/130°C fan/gas mark 2.
2 Arrange the tomatoes, cut-side up, in a small baking tin so they're sitting snugly next to each other.
3 Whisk together the olive oil, sherry vinegar, chopped thyme and rosemary in a bowl and season with salt and pepper. Spoon over the tomatoes, ensuring some of the chopped herbs land on top of each one. Roast in the oven for around 1 hour until they've slumped down to half their size.
4 Take out of the oven and drizzle with a little extra sherry vinegar while they're still warm.

SERVING SUGGESTION

Their juicy texture lends the tomatoes to being squished onto a thick slice of toast, tossed into freshly cooked pasta or tender new potatoes alongside lots of chopped herbs. They also make a dead simple starter if you partner them with a ball of mozzarella or its double-cream cousin, burrata – just remember to take either out of the fridge about half an hour before serving so that the flavour comes through. Serve half a ball of mozzarella or burrata each; be careful when slicing through the burrata as it will ooze everywhere, so you'll need a spoon to divvy it up. Lift onto a plate and spoon over a generous amount of the roasted tomatoes and top with a few basil or rocket leaves.

NOW TRY THIS...

Here's a quick pasta supper – a great one for those nights when you're pushed for time. It's enough for 4 people. Bring a large pan of water to the boil. Once boiling, stir in 400g conchiglie pasta and cook for 10–12 minutes until al dente – it should have a very slight bite to it.

Drain the pasta and tip it back into the pan with a tablespoon of the cooking water. Add a handful of chopped herbs or watercress, 4 chopped anchovies, around 10 chopped stoned olives, 1 teaspoon of red wine vinegar and a couple of tablespoons of the tomatoes. Season to taste, adding more vinegar if you need more acidity, then toss everything together and serve with a drizzle of extra virgin olive oil.

BRAISED LAMB WITH ROSEMARY AND RED WINE

Have you ever checked the seasoning of a casserole only to find it tastes a bit flat and needs something to bring all the flavours together? Stir in 1–2 teaspoons of sherry vinegar to sharpen it, leave for 5 minutes, then taste again to check the balance of flavour. Try this simple oven-braised recipe, scented with rosemary.

Serves 4

1 tbsp olive oil, plus extra for browning the meat

1 small red onion, chopped

1 celery stick, chopped

1 carrot, chopped

1 fat garlic clove, sliced

A sprig of rosemary

500g lamb shoulder, trimmed and cut into 2.5cm chunks

½ tbsp plain flour

125ml red wine

1–2 tsp sherry vinegar

1 Heat the oil in a large casserole pan and sauté the chopped onion, celery and carrot for 8–10 minutes until they start to soften and turn golden. Stir in the garlic and rosemary and cook for 1 minute. Scoop out and spoon into a large bowl.

2 Brown the meat – you can do this in two pans if you want to cook the meat more quickly. Put a frying pan and the casserole pan on the hob over a low–medium heat. Drizzle 1 teaspoon of oil into each pan and tip to swirl the oil over the bases. Add about six or seven pieces of meat to each pan

and leave them to brown on one side for a good minute or so, then turn them over – if they're not quite ready they'll still be stuck to the pan. Keep browning until they're all done, then spoon into the bowl with the vegetables.

3 Keep cooking the meat in batches, adding more oil as necessary, until you've browned it all. It's important to keep the pan over a low–medium heat so the juices on the bottom don't burn, otherwise the stew will taste bitter at the end.

4 Preheat the oven to 150°C/130°C fan/gas mark 2. Stir the flour into the pan and cook for 1–2 minutes until it starts to turn golden. Add the red wine and stir in, loosening any stuck bits on the base of the pan. Spoon the vegetable and meat mixture back into the pan then pour in enough hot water to just cover. Cover the pan with a lid and bring to a simmer. Transfer to the oven and cook for 2–2½ hours or until the meat is tender. Check every 40 minutes or so to make sure there's enough liquid covering the meat. Stir in the vinegar, check the seasoning and serve with creamy mash.

FIVE-HOUR PULLED PORK

Here's a recipe that needs very little work. Just marinate the pork then leave it to cook slowly in the oven until the meat can be pulled apart with two forks. The marinade turns lovely and caramelised on the outside as it cooks. There's a quick salsa to go with it at the end, too, with a sharpener of white wine vinegar to keep the other ingredients tasting oh so fresh. Serve with rice or sweet potatoes and a chopped salad.

900g pork shoulder, boned
4 garlic cloves, crushed
1 tsp each sea salt and freshly ground black pepper
2 tsp paprika
½ tsp ground cloves
2 tsp English mustard powder
3 tbsp white wine vinegar
A couple of splashes of Worcestershire sauce
1 tbsp tomato purée or sundried tomato paste
30g light muscovado sugar

1 First marinate the pork. Mix the garlic, salt, pepper and spices, mustard, vinegar, Worcestershire sauce, tomato purée or paste and sugar in a large sealable container. Add the pork and turn it over in the marinade to coat it. Cover and chill for up to a day.

2 When you want to cook it, take the pork out of the fridge around 30 minutes before it goes into the oven to bring it to room temperature. Turn the oven onto 150°C/130°C fan/ gas mark 2. Line the tin with baking parchment and put a

rack into it so that the pork isn't sitting on the base. Place the pork on the rack, then pour in 600ml water underneath it. Cover with foil. Cook in the oven for at least 5 hours. It's ready when the meat shreds easily.

FOR A QUICK ACCOMPANYING SALSA, TRY THIS

Slice the cheeks from 2 mangoes then criss-cross the fruit. Scoop out and into a bowl. Add a quarter of a red onion, finely chopped, and some chopped red chilli – start with half, then if it's not spicy enough, add more. Stir in 1 tablespoon of white wine vinegar, 1 teaspoon of light muscovado sugar and the zest and juice of 1 lime. Season with salt and stir well.

FATTY SAUSAGE?

Sounds like a medical affliction but it's not! If you've ever cooked bangers in a frying pan and find that instead of them glistening in a slick of oil, they're swimming in it, here's how to rescue them from tasting too fatty. Lift them onto a board and split each one open lengthways. Sprinkle with sherry vinegar (around 1 teaspoon per sausage) and grind over a little black pepper. Serve with a crisp just-washed salad (no need for any oil), crusty bread and dollop of creamy Dijon mustard on the side.

PORK VINDALOO

It's no surprise, bearing in mind its long history, that there are many variations of this Christian Goan dish. It's thought to be a riff on *carne de vinho e elhos*, the Portuguese dish which is a simple offering of pork cooked long and slow in wine vinegar and garlic until tender. Apparently the Portuguese brought chilli to India during the sixteenth century, but it wasn't until over 200 years or so later that this dish was rustled up there, born out of requests from the British for pork when they arrived in Southern India.

The vinegar serves two purposes here – it's used in the marinade so leaves the pork wonderfully tender, and it gives a sharpness to the curry gravy which stops it tasting too rich. The marinade, accompanying spices and ingredients used here to cook the meat have so much flavour that the only liquid called for is water (not stock). Serves 4 generously, with rice and naan on the side. Try it also with the pickled shallots on page 94. Any leftovers can be shredded and served cold in a naan with chopped lettuce, cucumber and tomatoes.

For the curry

1kg skinless shoulder of pork, chopped into 2–3cm pieces
3 tbsp vegetable oil
1 tsp mustard seeds
2 sprigs of curry leaves
2 onions, chopped
1 cinnamon stick
2 cardamom pods
6 garlic cloves, chopped

20g fresh ginger, chopped
2 green chillies, chopped
Sea salt and freshly ground black pepper

For the marinade

1 tsp cumin seeds
6 whole cloves
15 black peppercorns
1 red chilli, cut down the middle
1 tsp turmeric
6 garlic cloves, crushed
40g fresh ginger, grated
1½ tbsp tamarind paste
2 tbsp red wine vinegar
1 tsp salt
½ tbsp light muscovado sugar

1 First make the marinade by toasting the cumin, cloves and peppercorns in a small frying pan for 1–2 minutes until you can smell their aroma. Tip into a pestle and mortar and grind down to a powder. Tip into a sealable container and add the rest of the marinade ingredients. Stir everything together, add the pork and toss to coat in the marinade. Pop the lid on and marinate in the fridge for up to 8 hours.

2 Heat the oil in a large casserole pan over a medium heat and fry the mustard seeds and sprigs of curry leaves. As soon as they start to splutter, stir in the chopped onions, cinnamon stick and cardamom and season the mixture, then reduce the heat to low and cook for 10–12 minutes, stirring every

now and then until the onion starts to look translucent and turn golden on the edges. Stir in the garlic, ginger and green chillies and cook for 2–3 minutes.

3 Add the pork and any marinade to the pan and cook over a medium heat for 8–10 minutes, turning the pieces every now and then until golden on each side. Pour in 350ml hot water, season again, then cover with a lid. Bring to a simmer then turn the heat down to the lowest setting and simmer for 1 hour. After 30 minutes, give the curry a good stir. Replace the lid but keep stirring every now and then until the pork is tender. Check it around 10 minutes before the end and add 100–150ml hot water if the sauce looks dry.

LIGHTEN A CURRY

Whether it's a hot curry or a creamy dal you're serving alongside a simple bowl of steamed rice (or ordering from the takeaway!), try it with this refreshing pickle to sharpen the spicy flavours. Finely slice 1 small red onion or 2 large banana shallots and put in a bowl. Add 2 tablespoons of white wine vinegar and about ¼ teaspoon of finely crushed cumin seeds and coriander and ½ teaspoon each of salt and caster sugar. Add around 1 tablespoon of freshly chopped coriander then stir everything together and leave to marinate for 20 minutes before serving. It's punchy enough to clear blocked sinuses if you're suffering from a cold, too.

CHEAT'S CHICKEN TIKKA

Now this really is quicker than calling for a takeaway, and if you do a little bit of prep at breakfast time, it will be ready to go when you get in from work. The marinade is a humble marriage of store-cupboard ingredients, including tomato purée and spices, vinegar to tenderise the chicken and Greek yogurt to add a creamy flavour. Pick up some ready-made naan to grill or microwave on your way home and serve with sliced cucumber, red onion and tomatoes and you're all set.

Serves 4

1 tbsp tomato purée
1 tbsp medium curry powder
A good pinch of chilli powder
1 tbsp white wine vinegar
1 tsp olive oil
3cm piece of fresh ginger, peeled and grated
3 grated garlic cloves
30g Greek yogurt
½ tsp salt
¼ tsp freshly ground black pepper
500g chicken, cut into 2cm pieces

1 Put the tomato purée into a large bowl. Add the curry powder, chilli powder, vinegar, oil, ginger, garlic, yogurt, salt and pepper. Stir everything together.
2 Add the chicken to the bowl and toss well in the marinade. If you have time, set this aside for 20 minutes to seep into the chicken. (Or you can make it up to a day ahead, then

store it in a sealable container in the fridge until you want to cook it.)

3 When you're ready to cook, preheat the grill. Thread the marinated chicken onto skewers (if you're using bamboo, soak these first in warm water for 10–20 minutes). Lay the skewers on a lipped baking sheet, so the juices don't drip everywhere once they're cooked. Grill for 15 minutes without turning to get that slightly tandoor appearance on the outside (this will depend on how hot your grill is). To check they're cooked, cut through the thickest part of the meat to make sure no pink juices remain. Serve with rice.

AND HERE'S THE ALTERNATIVE TIKKA FOR VEGANS...

Use around 125g firm tofu (not the silken variety) per person and chop into 3cm cubes. Make the spiced marinade in a bowl as above, using the same quantity of coconut cream in place of the Greek yogurt, then stir in the tofu. Push onto skewers and grill for 5 minutes until golden and heated through.

DUCK WITH WALNUTS

There's tons of flavour in duck fat, but of course it's too rich to use on its own in a sauce. It needs something to cut through it. The vinegar used here – either red wine or Cabernet Sauvignon – works just like pouring red wine into a gravy by giving the sauce in this recipe its oomph. Keeping the pan over a medium heat and cooking the duck breasts skin-side down from the start releases quite a bit of fat but with it the rather delicious goodness – those sticky brown bits that'll be clinging to the base of the pan. Drain the fat off (see overleaf) then stir in nuts, the vinegar and orange juice for a touch of sweetness. Serve with blanched fresh peas, tossed with a handful of freshly chopped watercress and steamed new potatoes or crusty bread.

Serves 4

4 duck breasts, skin on
1½ tsp olive oil
30g chopped walnuts
Juice of 1 large orange
1 tbsp Cabernet Sauvignon red wine vinegar
A knob of butter (10–15g)
2 tbsp freshly chopped parsley

1   Score the skin of each duck breast (either slash it two or three times or work in a criss-cross pattern using a sharp knife). Put the oil in a large frying pan over a medium heat and cook the duck for 5 minutes to brown the skin. Lots of fat will have seeped out of the skin by the time it's lovely and golden.

2   Strain the fat into a bowl (chill and save to use for roasting potatoes) and turn the duck breasts over to the other side. Continue to cook for 10 minutes over a lowish heat until the duck breasts have cooked through and feel firm when you press the top with a knife.

3   Lift the breasts out into a bowl, cover and leave to rest. There should be a little fat left in the pan but not too much. Stir in the chopped walnuts and cook for a minute or two to toast them. Pour in the orange juice and red wine vinegar and bring to a simmer. Season well then add the knob of butter. Swirl around to melt the butter into the other ingredients, then simmer for a minute or two more to slightly thicken the sauce. Stir in the parsley.

4   Pour any of the rested juices into the pan and keep the pan over a low heat until the sauce has warmed through. Slice each duck breast and put on four warm plates. Spoon the sauce over the top and serve.

TO USE UP THAT LITTLE POT OF DUCK FAT...

You can store that little pot in the fridge for up to a month or freeze it. It'll give lots of flavour to roast potatoes or you can use it to sauté potatoes. Chop new potatoes into quarters and simmer until just tender. Drain well, add the fat to the pan then add the potatoes. Season with salt and cook until the potatoes are golden on the edges. Or spread the duck fat over a whole chicken before roasting – again, it gives additional flavour and will also help to crisp the skin of the finished bird.

THREE WAYS WITH RASPBERRY VINEGAR

Have you been given a bottle of raspberry vinegar but are short of ideas on how to use it? The sharp fruity flavour works well in both savoury and sweet offerings, as these three recipes demonstrate, but steer clear of fishy feasts. In the pizza, the flavour of the vinegar has an edge but works to offset the creamy cheese and slightly acidic tang of the tomatoes. In the starter it enhances the sweet fruit and musky flavour of the cured Italian ham, while in the pudding it works as a pin-sharp jolt to the tastebuds to offset the sweetness of the fruit and white chocolate.

ON PIZZA

Preheat the oven to the hottest setting and put a baking sheet in to heat up. Spread 1 tablespoon each of tomato purée over two large wholemeal Italian-style flatbreads. Slice 450g heritage tomatoes thinly and arrange over the top of the purée. Drizzle with a little oil and season well. Slide onto the preheated baking sheet and bake for 8–10 minutes until the flatbreads look crisp around the edge and the tomatoes have softened. Meanwhile, whisk 1½ tablespoons of raspberry vinegar and 1½ tablespoons of extra virgin olive oil together. Tear 150g ball buffalo mozzarella or burrata in half, then rip into rough pieces and scatter over the top of each pizza. Drizzle with the raspberry dressing and garnish with basil. Slice in half and serve each with a handful of rocket. Serves 4 for a light lunch.

IN A STARTER SALAD

Slice two ripe peaches or nectarines into thin wedges and arrange over a large platter. Scatter over a large handful of rocket. Nudge 6 slices of prosciutto crudo into the gaps and curl up slightly. Whisk 2 tablespoons of raspberry vinegar with ½ teaspoon of Dijon mustard and 1 tablespoon of extra virgin olive oil. Season well. Drizzle over the dressing then scatter over 1 tablespoon of toasted pine nuts. Serves 4 with a couple of breadsticks each.

TO DRESS A SUMMERY PUDDING

Slice 8 apricots in half and remove the kernels. Arrange, cut-side up, in a baking tray and dot each half with a smidgen of butter. Sprinkle 1 teaspoon of golden caster sugar over the whole lot. Grill for 5 minutes until golden and bubbling and the fruit is tender but still holds its shape. Arrange over a large platter and dot 125g raspberries in between the apricots. Spoon over 100g crème fraîche into little blobs all over. Whisk 1 tablespoon of raspberry vinegar together with the juice of ½ orange and ½ teaspoon of honey. Drizzle over the raspberry dressing and scatter over 1 tablespoon of toasted chopped pistachios and 2 squares of grated or chopped white chocolate. Serves 4.

RED PEPPER, CHICKPEA AND HARISSA DRESSING FOR PAN-FRIED HAKE

Sherry vinegar is made from the fortified wine, sherry, and has a slightly higher acidity than other vinegars, so it is an ideal match for sweet Mediterranean vegetables such as peppers. There's lots of flavour going on in this sauce, thanks to a dash of the spicy Moroccan chilli paste, harissa. The splash of sherry vinegar helps to cut through and enhance this when it's added at the end. You can make the dressing up to a day ahead; store it in the fridge in a sealable container. When it comes to serving, reheat the dressing in a pan gently, so the flavour of the vinegar doesn't cook away.

Serves 4

2 tbsp olive oil
1 red onion, chopped
2 red peppers, cut in half and deseeded
1 fat garlic clove, sliced
1 tsp harissa
400g can chickpeas, rinsed and drained
1 tbsp sherry vinegar
50–75ml water
Sea salt and freshly ground black pepper

1   Turn the grill onto the hottest setting. Heat the oil in a medium pan and stir in the onion. Season well and sauté over a very low heat for 10–15 minutes, stirring every now and then, until the onion has softened and is just starting to turn golden.

2   Meanwhile, set the peppers, cut-side down, on a baking sheet. Grill until the skins have almost all blackened then slide them into a bowl and cover (a pan lid is handy for this). Leave to steam for 5–10 minutes.

3   Stir the garlic and harissa into the onions and continue to cook for 2–3 minutes; take the pan off the heat.

4   Slide the skins off the peppers – if you're lucky they'll come off in one piece. Slice each half into thin strips and stir into the pan with the onions. Tip the chickpeas into the pan, then stir in the vinegar and water. Put the pan back on the heat and reheat gently. Check and adjust the seasoning just before serving with the pan-fried hake on the next page.

FOR THE PAN-FRIED HAKE

Serves 4

2 tbsp plain flour
A pinch of seasoning, such as a mix of paprika and smoked
*   paprika (optional)*
4 x 175g hake cutlets
1 tbsp olive oil
Knob of butter
Splash of sherry vinegar
Sea salt and freshly ground black pepper

1 Spoon the flour onto a plate and season well. Add the extra seasonings, if you like. Mix into the flour, then press the hake cutlets into the flour, turning them over so they're coated on both sides.

2 Heat the olive oil in a large frying pan over a medium heat. Lay the fish in the pan and cook for around 3 minutes on one side until dark golden. Turn over and cook the other side for a further 3 minutes.

3 Add a knob of butter to the pan and allow it to melt, then spoon the seasoned butter over each of the cutlets. Cook for another minute if necessary – the fish is ready when it easily comes away from the bone in the middle and can be flaked.

4 Splash a little sherry vinegar over the fish just before they're lifted out of the pan.

RECIPES

MULLET ESCABECHE

Cooking meat, fish or vegetable 'escabeche' is a Latin-based style of cuisine where the ingredient is partially cooked first, then finished in a hot cure containing vinegar. The dish is then left to cool while the vinegar works its magic and finishes off 'cooking' the ingredient. It's perfect for small fish such as mullet as it doesn't take long for the initial pan-frying. The dressing here is made from simple ingredients that you can switch up with whatever you have to hand. If you happen to have either saffron or paprika to hand, add a pinch to make it even more authentic.

Serves 2

75ml extra virgin olive oil, plus extra for frying
6 small, very fresh red mullet, scaled, gutted and cleaned
1 banana shallot, halved and finely sliced
1 tbsp pine nuts
1 tbsp sultanas
1 sprig of rosemary
4 tbsp red wine vinegar
Sea salt and freshly ground black pepper

1   Heat a little of the oil in a frying pan. Season the mullet and fry on each side for 2 minutes. Lay in a shallow dish or tray or sealable container.
2   Heat the 75ml oil in a pan until hot. Add the sliced shallot, pine nuts, sultanas and sprig of rosemary and heat for 2–3 minutes. Take the pan off the heat and stir in the vinegar.

3 Pour over the fish and cool. Serve with steamed greens and potatoes, roughly crushed, seasoned and tossed with a knob of butter. The potatoes should be soft enough to fluff up when shaken in the colander and they'll also absorb the moreish dressing from the fish.

STUFFED COURGETTES – ASIAN-STYLE

A glut of homegrown vegetables is both a gardener's delight and despair – it's brilliant to have grown so much successfully but how to find yet another inventive way to use up the crop? Here's a twist on an old favourite that calls for very little prep, leaving the oven to do all the work. Stuffing courgettes and roasting until tender is a grand way of making the most of them, as all of the soft middle is used too, and provides both a stronger taste and texture to the filling. Instead of more traditional Mediterranean-style flavours, this recipe calls for a handful of Asian ingredients – shallots, ginger, lemongrass and fragrant coriander and basil – with smoked mackerel and finishes it with rice vinegar to cut through the richness. There's plenty going on here, so if you want a side, serve it with some plain noodles, tossed in a little oil to stop them sticking.

Serves 2

800g courgettes (about 2 large overblown summer ones)
1 tbsp sunflower oil, plus extra to drizzle
1 banana shallot, finely chopped
2cm piece fresh ginger, chopped
1 lemongrass stalk, chopped
1 red or green chilli, deseeded and chopped
2 cherry plum tomatoes, chopped
1 tbsp rice vinegar
2 smoked mackerel fillets (around 130g), skinned
2 tbsp freshly chopped coriander, plus extra to garnish
1 tbsp freshly chopped Thai basil, plus extra to garnish
½ lime, halved

1   Preheat the oven to 200°C/180°C fan/gas mark 6. Slice each courgette in half through the stalk and use a spoon to scoop out the soft middle. Discard any seeds – they won't cook down and will be tough to eat – then chop the flesh.

2   Heat the oil in a medium pan over a medium heat and stir in the shallot, ginger, lemongrass, chilli and chopped flesh of the courgette. Sauté for about 5 minutes until softened and starting to turn golden.

3   Stir in the tomatoes and vinegar and continue to cook for a minute or two more, then turn off the heat. Flake the mackerel, add to the pan along with the chopped herbs and season again.

4   Season the inside of each courgette and drizzle with a little oil. Divide the mixture evenly between the courgettes then drizzle 1 tablespoon of water over each half. Roast in the oven for 20 minutes until the courgette is tender. Garnish with a few extra sprigs of herbs and serve with a wedge of lime.

SALADS

You may have just a handful of rocket or spinach or a Little Gem lettuce to hand, but with an expertly mixed dressing, they can be transformed into a worthy side. Think one part vinegar to three parts oil for the most basic combination. Pair with a simple griddled steak, an everyday plate of poached eggs on toast or a crisp-skinned piece of pan-fried fish. Read on for extra ideas…

3 CLASSIC (ISH) SALADS AND THEIR DRESSINGS

Sometimes the most simple marriages of ingredients are the most rewarding. Knowing how to knock up a great salad means you'll never be short of supper ideas on those nights when time is short and all that's to hand is a jumble of ingredients. Slicing, dicing and chopping them into uniform-sized pieces and tossing in an aromatic dressing will transform even the most unlikely random variety. The ratio of vinegar to oil will depend on the ingredients you are gathering and will vary from one part to four or a third of vinegar to oil or half and half. It's worth experimenting and tasting as you go to find out what you like best. Here are three favourite dressings plus a suggested salad in which to use them – just vary the main parts according to what you have in.

FRENCH

Pour 4 tablespoons of olive oil (see recipe tip below) into a jar, 1 tablespoon of red wine vinegar, 1 teaspoon of Dijon mustard (or use ½ teaspoon of English mustard if you only have that to hand) and 1 crushed garlic clove; season with salt and freshly ground black pepper then secure the lid and shake well. If you find the Dijon hasn't properly blended with the other ingredients, add 1 teaspoon of boiling water and shake again to dissolve it.

Serve with...

This riff on a Niçoise salad. Start by cooking the potatoes. Bring a medium pan of water to the boil. Cut 350g new potatoes into 2cm cubes by halving and quartering them through the length then chopping them once or twice again across the body. Cook in the pan for 8 minutes until you can stick the point of a sharp knife through them. After 2 minutes of cooking, add 2 large room-temperature eggs and cook for 6 minutes. After another 2 minutes, add 100g green beans, trimmed and chopped, and cook until tender. Drain everything well through a colander and rinse under cold running water. Set the colander aside and prepare the main salad ingredients.

Separate the leaves of 2 Little Gem lettuces, cutting the large pieces in half to even them out. Put them in a large wide salad bowl or spread over a flat platter and spoon over the cooled potatoes and beans. Next, top with 2 tomatoes, cut into wedges, 3 or 4 pieces of marinated pepper, cut into thin slivers, and a couple of spoonfuls of pitted olives.

Crack the shells of the boiled eggs and cut the eggs in half – the yolks will be firm with a slightly runny centre – and put them on top along with the tuna from a small tin (around 120g) of tuna preserved in oil (use the oil for the dressing – see above), then scatter over some freshly chopped parsley. Drizzle over the dressing and serve. Plenty for four people, especially if you add bread, too.

ITALIAN

Put 3 tablespoons of olive oil, 1½ tablespoons of white or traditional balsamic vinegar, 1 halved garlic clove and a sprig of basil into a jar; season with salt and freshly ground black pepper then secure the lid and shake well.

Serve with...

A heap of washed rocket (around 50g), 200g halved cherry tomatoes and 125g small mozzarella balls (either *bocconcini* or *perle*/pearls – drained weight). The role of the basil and garlic is just to impart their flavour into the oil and vinegar, so strain them out before using the dressing. Serves 4 with squares of focaccia or fingers of ciabatta.

GREEK

Pour 4 tablespoons of extra virgin olive oil into a jar and add 2 tablespoons of red wine vinegar, 2 teaspoons of freshly chopped oregano; season with salt and freshly ground black pepper then secure the lid and shake well.

Serve with...

Quarter six ripe and juicy tomatoes, then put them into a salad bowl. Add ½ cucumber, halved, deseeded and sliced into half-moons. Throw in around 50g Kalamata olives and 1 small sliced red onion. Pour over half the dressing and toss well. Put a 200g slab of feta cheese in the middle, spoon over the remaining dressing and let everyone dig into the cheese to divvy it up with the salad vegetables. Serve with warm pitta bread or those wonderful sesame-topped breadsticks.

A SIMPLE COUSCOUS SALAD

This recipe calls for half a standard 500g packet of couscous, so you're left with exactly the right amount to make this again! It's a good foil for rich-tasting roasted vegetables, a Middle-Eastern spiced meat, fish or vegetable tagine, or as a base for a salad box. Just add chickpeas, chopped tomatoes, peppers and crumbled feta for a very quick lunch. Also try adding past-their-best oranges – the ones that have languished in the fruit bowl for a while and have slightly dry skin and give when squeezed. These are particularly useful here as the juice tastes slightly sweeter.

Serves 2

For the couscous

250g couscous
275ml boiling water

For the dressing

Juice of 2 small oranges
1½ tbsp sherry vinegar
1 tbsp extra virgin olive oil
50g toasted pine nuts
¼ tsp each salt and freshly ground black pepper
Handful of chopped coriander or parsley

1   Put the couscous into a large heatproof bowl, then pour over the boiling water and cover with a pan lid or a plate. Leave to steam for 10 minutes.

2   For the dressing, pour the orange juice into a separate bowl then add the sherry vinegar, extra virgin olive oil, pine nuts and salt and pepper. Toss in the chopped coriander or parsley.

3   Once the couscous has finished steaming and all the water has been absorbed, fork it through to fluff up the grains. Pour over the dressing and stir everything again. Eat immediately or store in a sealable container in the fridge for up to four days.

RED WINE VINEGAR ADDS ZING TO AN ITALIAN SALAD

Bread goes stale more quickly in the summer, so if you have a chunk of ciabatta or sourdough that feels as heavy and dry as a brick, use it in panzanella. It's an Italian classic from the region of Tuscany whereby stale chunks are soaked in water to soften them until they feel like a wet sponge. If you're not a fan of soggy bread, this alternative, where the tomatoes are marinated with the dressing to allow the juices to seep out first, before the bread is added, keeps more of a bite to the chunks. Key to this recipe is the red wine vinegar – it softens the sharp taste of the red onion and also brings out the juices in the tomato.

Serves 4 alongside other salads for a barbecue

6 ripe tomtaoes
¼ red onion, chopped
2 tbsp red wine vinegar
150g stale bread
2 tbsp extra virgin olive oil
2 sprigs basil, roughly torn
Sea salt and freshly ground black pepper

1 Chop the tomatoes into chunks and put in a bowl with the chopped onion and vinegar. Season well and set aside for 10 minutes.

2 Chop the bread into chunks and stir into the tomatoes with the olive oil and the torn basil. Set aside to soak for a further 10 minutes before serving.

AND FOR THE TOTALLY INAUTHENTIC VERSION...

For a quick-to-prep lunch to take to work, use that stale chunk of bread in this. The half-and-half ratio of vinegar to oil keeps the whole salad tasting fresh. Spoon a couple of tablespoons of leftover chopped roasted vegetables in a sealable container (or two, three or four pots if you're making for more). Layer the following on top: chopped fresh tomatoes, a small piece of chopped cucumber, a couple of tablespoons of chickpeas, some mozzarella pearls or chopped cheese, a few torn basil leaves, a little chopped rocket and a chunk of chopped stale bread. Whisk together ½ tablespoon each of extra virgin olive oil and red wine vinegar per person and season well. Pour over the top then seal the lid. Admiration from work colleagues guaranteed.

MAKING THE MOST OF PRESERVED TUNA

Good-quality preserved tuna – the sort that's jarred or tinned in olive oil, perhaps with some seasonings or herbs – really is a store-cupboard saviour. You'll find a much wider range in European delis and supermarkets, so stock up on tins of other preserved fish while you're there.

Here are two recipes to keep in your arsenal. First up is a universal salad that's simple enough for a quick weekend lunch or as a starter for a relaxed supper with friends. Make sure there's enough crusty bread to go round to mop up the dressing. Then there's a pâté – tuna blitzed in minutes in the blender with spring onions, herbs and yogurt – which can be served on hot toast with soup or spooned into Little Gem lettuce leaves, sprinkled with some non-pareilles capers (the tiny ones) and more chopped herbs.

FOR A SALAD THAT SERVES FOUR

First make the dressing. Drain the oil from two 120g cans of tuna into a small bowl and add 2 tablespoons of red or white wine vinegar, 1 finely chopped tomato (deseed it first if you have the inclination and/or time) and a small handful of finely chopped parsley. Season well, tasting as you go. You may want to add a little more vinegar depending on the balance of flavour.

Shred 1 medium mooli radish into ribbons (use a spiraliser if you have one or a serrated Y-peeler) then do the same with ½ cucumber, scraping out the seeds if you're not keen on them. Halve and deseed 1 red pepper, then slice it into thin strips. Mix all the vegetables in a large salad bowl.

Spoon the dressing over the salad, toss together and flake over the tuna.

FOR THE QUICK TUNA PÂTÉ

Trim 2 spring onions, then chop them roughly and put them in a mini blender with 1 tablespoon of cider vinegar. Swirl the blender bowl around so the vinegar soaks into the pieces. Drain and reserve the oil from a 120g can of tuna then add the fish to the bowl with 1 tablespoon of reserved oil, 1 tablespoon of non-pareille capers and small handful of roughly chopped parsley. Blitz until smooth, adding more oil if you want a looser texture. Taste and season before serving. You can save the rest of the oil for roasting vegetables or to use as a base for a pasta sauce.

DIPS AND SAUCES

With a bottle of vinegar to hand, it's possible to make a super-instant side to heighten all sorts of wonderful delights. Swap ketchup for this uber-quick, measure-and-stir dip to serve alongside a bowlful of chips. Or partner it with a heap of dill and a spike of mustard in a sauce. Simple and effective, this transforms a plate of smoked fish into a decadent feast. These and other tricks will form part of your recipe arsenal for years to come.

QUICK DILL SAUCE FOR SMOKED FISH

You really do need a touch of acidity with cured and smoked fish, whether it's squeezing the juice from a wedge of lemon over the top or drizzling over a dressing made with vinegar – it cuts through the fatty richness of the flesh and will soften any overly smoky morsels.

Serve this sauce with a selection of fish – smoked mackerel (peppered or plain), brown shrimp or crayfish, and ribbons of smoked salmon (look out for the pink-tinged, beetroot-cured offering – it always sparks a conversation). This crowd-pleasing, no-effort starter, once you've made the dressing, really is just an assembly job.

For the dill sauce

10g dill sprigs
1 tbsp olive oil
2 tsp English mustard
½ tsp golden caster sugar
1 tbsp white wine vinegar
Sea salt and freshly ground black pepper

To serve

A selection of smoked fish (about 100g per person), see intro
Sprigs of watercress, endive fingers or Little Gem leaves

1   First make the sauce. In a small food processor, put the dill, olive oil, mustard, sugar, vinegar and 1 tablespoon of water. Season well and blend until smooth. It'll be bright yellow with dashes of the dill cut through it. The sauce can be made up to two days ahead, then stored in the fridge.

2   When you're ready to serve, arrange the smoked fish on a large platter. Remove the skin from the mackerel, then gently tease apart the flesh into big chunks with a fork. Add spoonfuls of the brown shrimp and/or crayfish, then tuck curls of smoked salmon ribbons among the spaces. Pepper any empty spots of the platter with little handfuls of watercress and fingers of endive or Little Gem lettuce and serve drizzled with the sweet dill sauce.

HOMEMADE HOISIN-STYLE SAUCE

This may not be a totally authentic representation of the classic Asian dip but it's pretty quick and made mostly out of store-cupboard ingredients – the sort you'll have in, that is – so it won't leave you with lots of bits and pieces that you don't use again. The vinegar serves to thin the sauce down while its flavour cuts through and softens the sweetness of the other ingredients.

Makes enough for 2 servings in a stir-fry or dip

3 tbsp smooth peanut butter
2 tbsp dark soy sauce
1 tsp tomato purée
¼ tsp Chinese five spice (optional)
¼ tsp ground white pepper
1 tbsp rice vinegar
1 tbsp chopped salted peanuts

1 Put the peanut butter, soy sauce, tomato purée, five spice and white pepper into a bowl. Pour the vinegar over the top and stir together until smooth.

2 Use this in a stir-fry, then sprinkle over the salted peanuts at the end. Or, for a dipping sauce, spoon into a bowl and sprinkle with the salted peanuts before serving.

A SOFTER-TASTING AIOLI FOR PAN-FRIED FISH

Garlic mayo, otherwise known as aioli, is simply made with egg yolks, garlic and olive oil. Here a splash of vinegar is also added at the end to stop the sauce tasting too oily. The garlic is cooked lightly at the beginning so it gives a softer flavour than the traditional recipe

Makes enough to serve 8

250ml olive oil
2 garlic cloves, thickly sliced
3 large egg yolks
2–3 tsp sherry vinegar
Sea salt

1 Put 1 tablespoon of the oil into a small frying pan and heat gently. Stir in the garlic cloves and cook for about 30 seconds – just until they've softened and are about to turn golden. If they cook for any longer the cut sides will go crispy and they'll be harder to mash into the oil. Take the pan off the heat and mash the garlic into the oil.

2 Put the egg yolks into a medium bowl and whisk a little – use a balloon whisk if you dare (though there's no doubt about it – your arm will start to ache halfway through and you may be calling for help) or go straight for the electric hand whisk (much easier!). Add a drop of the olive oil and whisk in.

3 Continue, adding a little more oil each time and whisking between each drizzle, until the mixture starts to thicken and emulsify. At this stage, about halfway, you should be able to

add the oil in a more or less constant stream while whisking. If it looks as though the mixture is about to split, stop adding the oil and whisk vigorously on the highest speed, which should keep the mixture together (see note below).

4   Once all the oil has been added, whisk in the mashed garlic and 1–2 teaspoons of the sherry vinegar (or to taste) and season with salt. This will keep in a clean jar stored in the fridge for up to four days. Once chilled it's more like a spread and is also great on a toasted sandwich.

TWO POINTS TO NOTE HERE...

If you fancy using extra virgin olive oil here, the colour of the aioli will be much darker, with a green tinge. It will have a stronger olive oil flavour, too, so experiment with the quantity of vinegar you add as it will soften the taste. For a lighter flavour and colour, use half each of light olive oil and sunflower oil.

If the aioli does split, first whisk in 1–2 teaspoons boiling water to stabilise the mixture. If that doesn't work, you'll need to start again with another egg yolk. Put it into a separate clean bowl, whisk to break it down, then add the split mixture, a spoonful at a time, and whisk in until all of it has been added. Finish off the recipe as in step 4.

HOW TO USE UP LEFTOVER EGG WHITES

As this recipe only uses the yolks, rather than waste the whites you can use them for the Golden Pavlova on page 148, or they freeze well, as do yolks. Store the egg white in a clean grease-free pot (if there's a speck of oiliness in the pot the whites won't whisk to their full volume), seal, label and freeze for up to one month. If you're freezing yolks, whisk lightly in a small sealable pot and sprinkle with a pinch of salt first, then seal, label and again freeze for up to one month.

ONE-MINUTE DIPS FOR CHIPS

Ditch the tomato ketchup and try one of these with hot chips instead. Each recipe makes enough for 2.

DIP ONE

Spoon 2 tablespoons of ready-made mayonnaise into a small bowl and stir in 2 teaspoons of balsamic vinegar. This is particularly good made with those slightly cheaper mayos (those with added sugar) as the acidity balances the overall taste. Also delicious with nuggets of crispy sautéed potatoes.

DIP TWO

Spoon 2 tbsp crème fraiche, 1 tsp Dijon mustard and 2 tsp cider vinegar into a bowl. Season and add 1 tbsp freshly chopped parsley. Stir together and serve. Season the chips first with smoked paprika along with sea salt for extra flavour. This is also fantastic with sausages or drizzle over sausage and mash as an alternative to gravy.

A CANNY TIP TO STRETCH AN AVOCADO TO FEED A FEW MORE...

Whizzing avocado with yogurt produces a very moreish, moussey texture in this dip and is an instant way to make just one piece of fruit go a bit further. Adding the vinegar gives it a lovely sharp taste. Using paprika, cumin and coriander, with their musky Middle Eastern notes, may sound like an unusual match but they work really well here. Serve with fingers of toasted brown pitta bread, sticks of carrot and pepper and trimmed radishes. Serves 4–6.

To make it, simply cut a medium avocado in half and whip out the stone. Spoon all of the flesh into a mini blender and add 50g full-fat Greek yogurt, ½ tablespoon of red wine vinegar, ¼ teaspoon each of paprika, ground cumin and coriander. Whiz until smooth, then season to taste with salt and freshly ground black pepper.

DIPPING SAUCE FOR SPRING ROLLS AND DUMPLINGS

This is a simple three-ingredient mix of soy sauce (so there's no need for extra salt), Chinese vinegar (which has a wonderful smoky taste and cuts through the soy) and chilli oil. You can make this in whatever quantities you need for however many people. Use around 1 teaspoon each of Chinese vinegar and soy sauce per person and pour into a little dipping bowl. Add a splash of chilli oil – or as much as you dare – to season with a kick of spice and heat.

ALTERNATIVE DIPPING SAUCE

This is easy to scale up or down, depending on how many you're serving. For each person, put 1 tsp rice vinegar, 1 tsp mirin rice wine, a pinch of sugar and 1 tsp chopped salted peanutes into a bowl. Add a little chopped red chilli and a few slices of garlic. Season with salt and stir. This is also a really good dressing for rice noodles.

ALSO TRY CHINESE VINEGAR IN THIS...

Leftover gravy? Don't bin it — even if it's just a couple of spoonfuls. Keep it in a sealed container for up to five days in the fridge. It is also really good as a base sauce in a stir-fry with a splash of smoky Chinese vinegar to accentuate the sweetness of the stir-fried veg. Use 150-200g sliced vegetables per person (white cabbage, carrots, red, white or spring onions, peppers and beans are all good with sliced ginger and garlic). Heat around 1 tablespoon of oil in a large wok and stir-fry for a few minutes until the vegetables are starting to turn golden. Stir in the jellied gravy and watch it melt, then add 1 teaspoon of Chinese vinegar, 1 teaspoon of soy sauce and 1 teaspoon of sesame oil. Season with salt and white pepper and toss again, cooking for a few more minutes. Taste and adjust the seasoning, adding more soy as necessary. Sprinkle with sesame seeds before serving.

You can also try using leftover gravy in a risotto, with shredded meat and lots of Parmesan stirred in at the end. Or toss it with drained pasta, finished with a knob of butter. Either way, make sure you add a splash of balsamic vinegar at the end to provide a contrast to the rich Parmesan and buttery juices.

CLASSIC DRESSING FOR OYSTERS

This is quite often referred to as a shallot dressing, but the classic name for this in French is *sauce mignonette*, so-called because mignonette used to be the name for a sachet of spices used in stocks and soups. But latterly it's become culinary shorthand in kitchen French for cracked black pepper. It takes minutes to put together but the vinegar here gives a real zing to the saline, sometimes creamy, taste of oysters.

FOR EVERY 6 OYSTERS, MAKE UP THIS DRESSING:

Finely chop 2 regular shallots or 1 banana shallot (the long thin ones) and put in a bowl with 2 tablespoons of red wine vinegar. Season with freshly ground black pepper and keep at room temperature until ready to serve.

SNACKS AND NIBBLES

Nothing beats a homemade savoury treat in our book… whether it's a bite-size morsel to sop up a glass of booze, something to satisfy those peckish moments before supper or a lighter-than-normal sit-down meal. Here's a collection of super-easy ideas – try spiced nuts with tahini and honey or no-fry crisps – both are quick to rustle up from a handful of ingredients. There's also a mushroom toast topper with a dash of vinegar to add a touch of acidity to the rich flavour.

DRINKS NIBBLES

Offering something round at the same time as touting that first drink of the evening is a must as it helps to slow the alcohol being absorbed and most importantly stops you from feeling tiddly too quickly! The next three recipes are rustled up from store-cupboard stalwarts and take very little effort at all. Each one serves 4 alongside other nibbles.

HOT SALT AND VINEGAR CRISPS

This is a twist on serving crisps and uses just a couple of new potatoes. Don't worry, there's no call for a deep-fat fryer here, as these are done in the oven until the little rounds are golden and baked through then seasoned with salt and, of course, splashed with vinegar at the end to lift their flavour.

Serves 4

100g unpeeled new potatoes
½ tbsp olive oil
1 tbsp sherry vinegar
Sea salt

1   Preheat the oven to 200°C/180°C fan/gas mark 6. Slice the potatoes thinly – about 1mm thick. A mandolin or food processor is good for this. Put into a bowl with the olive oil and a pinch of salt. Toss well.

2   Line a tray with baking parchment (not greaseproof paper) and spread the slices over so they're in one layer. Bake for 10 minutes, then flip each one over and bake for a further 5 minutes.

3   Sprinkle with the vinegar and return to the oven for a further 1–2 minutes for it to soak into the rounds and warm through. Watch them carefully as they can burn very quickly as soon as you turn your back. Slide the crisps off the parchment and into bowls and serve straightaway.

CUMIN-SPICED NUTS

These spiced nuts combine musky cumin, tahini and a touch of vinegar and honey for a luxurious-tasting nibble. The vinegar brings all the ingredients together to make a bowlful that's so much more than the sum of its parts.

Serves 4

100g mixed nuts
1 tbsp tahini
1 tbsp honey
2 tsp cider vinegar
1 tsp cumin seeds
Sea salt and freshly ground black pepper

1 Preheat the oven to 200°C/180°C fan/gas mark 6. Tip the nuts into a bowl and add the tahini, honey, vinegar and cumin seeds. Season well with salt and pepper. Stir everything together so the nuts are well coated with the spiced sticky sauce.

2 Spread out on a tray lined with baking parchment and roast for 10 minutes until golden. Leave to cool before serving.

CHILLI-SPICED OLIVES

This last nibble comes courtesy of a jar of olives in brine. They're marinated in a homemade concoction of olive oil and red wine vinegar that brings a fruity taste to the marinade, as well as a hint of chilli and lemon. It's very simple, but very effective.

Serves 4

300–350g jar Kalamata olives in brine
1 tbsp olive oil
2 tsp red wine vinegar
Pinch of chilli flakes
1 tsp lemon zest
Sea salt

1   Drain the olives and tip into a bowl. Stir in the oil, vinegar, chilli flakes, lemon zest and a good pinch of salt.
2   Set aside to marinate for at least an hour if serving on the same day, or store in the fridge in an airtight container (or use the rinsed-out jar) for up to five days.

THE BEAUTY OF BALSAMIC

Back in the 90s it was *de rigueur* to serve a small dish of olive oil and balsamic vinegar with bread at the beginning of every restaurant meal. It became so popular (and we were so addicted to it, too) that even those places that weren't serving *cucina rustica Italiana* would offer it. It may have dropped off the culinary agenda slightly now but Italians still love to serve balsamic in numerous ways...

WITH FINGERS OF FENNEL

This makes a nice alternative to hunks of bread. Slice ½ fennel bulb in half through the root and cut away the core. Then slice the rest of it, still cutting lengthways, into finger-sized pieces. Spoon 2 tablespoons of good extra virgin olive oil and 1 tablespoon of balsamic vinegar into a small dish. The one-part vinegar to two of olive oil provides the right balance of acidity to the slightly fruity-flavoured fennel. Arrange the fennel fingers on a plate to serve with the dip.

DOTTED OVER CARPACCIO

This tricolore salad – red from the wafer-thin slices of raw beef fillet, white from shaved Parmesan and green from rocket leaves – is wonderfully simple to prepare. Wrap the tubular fillet (anything from 5cm upwards) in cling film then freeze until firm. Take off the cling film and use a very sharp knife to slice the beef fillet into thin rounds. Arrange each piece, slightly overlapping, on a large platter. Scatter over some rocket and top with shavings of Parmesan cheese. Drizzle a little balsamic vinegar over the top and season with freshly ground black pepper before serving. If you can, use the syrupy and slightly sweeter variety of balsamic for this and just trickle it over. It'll provide a foil to the peppery bite of the rocket.

SERVED WITH STEAK

Simply plonk a bottle on the table straight after your just-over-the-coals slab of meat has been presented. Again, the good syrupy variety, drizzled over sparingly, is wonderful here to bring out the flavours of the meat.

AS PART OF A THREE-INGREDIENT SALAD

A favourite in Bologna, this comprises the leaves of bitter red chicory, grilled mortadella (the baby-pink cured pork sausage dotted with white spots of pork fat) and just a drizzle of balsamic vinegar over the top. The sweet flavour of the balsamic counteracts the bitterness of the chicory, while the fatty mortadella adds the essential meaty flavour.

TO SEASON TORTELLONI

Cook a batch of ricotta-based tortelloni and drain well. Return to the pan with a knob of butter and some finely grated Parmesan and season well. Spoon among plates and drizzle over balsamic vinegar before serving. Just like salt and pepper, this acidic seasoning should only be a little addition as it serves as a high note to the other ingredients rather than a major player.

MUSHROOM TOAST TOPPER

However you're cooking mushrooms, it's essential for oil or butter to come into play. Don't even contemplate simmering them in water or they'll end up as soggy as a wet dishcloth. This recipe calls for both oil and butter and the mushrooms are seasoned well to maximise their flavour. A splash of balsamic at the end is used to enhance the earthiness, then they're blitzed with cream cheese to create that all-important smooth texture.

Depending on which variety of mushrooms you use here, you'll end up with a mixture that appears dove grey in colour, or a topping that's resolutely black and looks like charcoal. No matter, it's still delicious and also doubles up as a great pâté for a pre-dinner appetiser. Serve on crostini – those crisp little rounds of bread cut from a baguette and baked or toasted – then sprinkle with a little freshly chopped parsley or chives.

Serves 2

100g chopped mushrooms, with stalks
1½ tsp olive oil
1½ tsp butter
1 garlic clove, crushed
1 tsp balsamic vinegar
40g cream cheese
2–4 slices good-quality bread
25g Parmesan
Sea salt and freshly ground black pepper

1 Heat the olive oil and butter in a pan. Once the butter has melted, stir in the mushrooms and season well. Cook for 5 minutes, stirring often, until the mushrooms have wilted down. Stir in the garlic clove and cook for a further 2 minutes. Then turn off the heat and stir in the balsamic vinegar.

2 Tip the mixture into a small food processor and blend until smooth. Add the cream cheese and blitz again. Taste to check the seasoning and adjust accordingly.

3 Preheat the grill. Toast the bread on one side and then turn it over and spread the mixture on top. Use a fine grater to cover the top with Parmesan or another strong-flavoured hard cheese. Grill until melted and bubbling. Serve with black pepper and a trickle of balsamic over the top.

SHERRY VINEGAR MUSHROOMS

The small, closed-cup mushrooms (either white or chestnut) are good for this recipe. If they're tiddlers, leave them whole then slice the rest in half so they're all evenly sized. Mushrooms are similar to aubergines when cooking, in that their sponge-like texture will soak up any oil or butter that comes their way, so resist adding any more even if you think the pan looks dry. As they bubble away, the heat will bring out their natural juices and finish off cooking them. For the dressing, add a good knob of butter and the all-essential vinegar to give that sour taste that balances the buttery juices.

Serves 2–4

300g mushrooms
1 tbsp olive oil
15g butter
1½ tbsp sherry vinegar
½ tsp thick-set honey
1 tbsp fresh parsley, chopped
Sea salt and freshly ground black pepper

1 Heat the olive oil in a heavy-based saucepan, add the mushrooms and cover the pan with a lid. Cook over a low–medium heat for 5 minutes, shaking the pan every now and then until the mushrooms start to look golden.

2 Add the butter, vinegar and honey, season well and cover again. Cook for 1–2 minutes to make a sauce. Taste for seasoning and adjust accordingly. Serve sprinkled with the parsley alongside a chunk of bread or steamed basmati rice.

DESSERTS

Sweet things may not be the first thought for a culinary use of vinegar but its acidic quality works in surprising ways... For example, a dash of balsamic vinegar in the well-loved and simple Italian recipe for *fragole all'aceto balsamico* heightens the flavour of summer strawberries, or add a spoonful of white wine vinegar to egg whites to help create a chemical reaction and stabilise them in the mallowy confection that is pavlova.

SWEET RASPBERRY VINEGAR FOR ICE CREAM AND DRINKS

It may sound weird to add vinegar to make a sweet cordial but actually this really works. The Cabernet Sauvignon vinegar brings just the right amount of acidity to this, without it tasting too cloying. It's great drizzled over plain vanilla ice cream and also perks up a lower-budget sparkling wine, such as Crémant de Loire. You can also dilute it with sparkling water and add lots of ice for a refreshing cooler. This recipe makes around 100ml; store in the fridge for up to a week and use around 1 tablespoon per serving.

Put 150g raspberries into a medium pan. Pour in the juice of half an orange, 50g golden caster sugar and 50ml Cabernet Sauvignon red wine vinegar. Place the pan over a medium heat and use a potato masher to mash the raspberries into the mixture. Heat until the sugar has dissolved then increase the heat to a simmer and cook for 5 minutes. Keep mashing the mixture to press out all the juice from the fruit.

Strain through a sieve and into a bowl. Stir the fruit pulp with a wooden spoon to make sure you've extracted all the liquid – don't forget to scrape the underside of the sieve to get this bit in too. Stir well. Pour into a sterilised jar (see page 157), cool and chill.

BRING OUT THE SWEETNESS IN STRAWBERRIES

Fragole all'aceto balsamico is a classic Italian dessert from Emilia-Romagna that calls for a splash of good-quality syrupy balsamic vinegar to be poured over ripe strawberries. If you have a more liquid (and cheaper) version, try this delicious but slightly unorthodox treatment instead: stir 1 teaspoon of vinegar with 1 teaspoon of maple syrup in a medium bowl. Add 250g sliced strawberries and toss them in the dressing. Set aside at room temperature for 15–20 minutes to allow the flavours to mingle together. This makes enough to serve four spooned over a ball of good vanilla ice cream.

PEACHES WITH VERJUS AND ROSEMARY

This is a sumptuous summer pudding that can be served warm or chilled, and it is its simplicity that makes it such a perfect ending to a meal. The softer quality of verjus, which is made from raisins, is a perfect match for the fruity flavours that come through in the syrup here. There are just four ingredients so it really is very simple to make and can be prepared up to three days ahead if you want, and served chilled.

Serves 4

100g golden caster sugar
1 bushy sprig of rosemary, plus a few more to garnish (optional)
4 peaches
100ml verjus

1 Pour the sugar into a medium pan and add 500ml water and the sprig of rosemary. Heat gently to dissolve the sugar. Add the whole peaches and cover the pan with a lid. Simmer for 10 minutes until they are soft. Lift them out carefully using a slotted spoon and set on a plate to cool.

2 Pour the verjus into the pan and bring to the boil. Turn the heat down a little and simmer for 5 minutes until the syrup has reduced by half.

3 Carefully skin the peaches. Cut around the stone and carefully lift each half away from it. Put two halves into each bowl then strain the syrup over the top, garnish with extra rosemary and serve.

AN EXTRA TIP TO USE AS A STARTER...

This dish can double up as a starter if you continue to simmer the syrup until it's reduced to about a quarter of its volume. Skin the peaches as above and arrange one or two halves on each plate – quantities depend on entirely what else you are serving and eating here. Slide a couple of pieces of blue cheese onto each plate, too, along with a small handful of rocket and season with salt and freshly ground black pepper. Drizzle over a little extra virgin olive oil and serve with soft bread such as ciabatta to mop up the sauce.

CHOCOLATE SHARING MOUSSE WITH BLUEBERRIES AND PECANS

A splash of honey vinegar plus a handful of tart blueberries and pecans stops this confection tasting too sweet. If you have any ground cinnamon to hand, sprinkle it over just before serving, too. Quick note: if you're serving this to vegans, check the ingredients list on the chocolate packet first to make sure it isn't made with milk, and swap the honey for maple syrup and the honey vinegar for cider vinegar.

Serves 4

80g dark chocolate (at least 60% cocoa solids), broken up into small pieces
1 tsp honey
2 tsp honey vinegar
Around 150ml aquafaba (drained chickpea water)
A handful of blueberries
10g chopped pecan nuts

1 Put the dark chocolate and honey into a large bowl and melt on low in the microwave for 4 minutes, checking every 30 seconds. Shake the bowl every now and then to make sure the chocolate isn't overheating and is melting evenly. Cool.

2 Wipe a glass bowl with a little bit of the vinegar. Pour the chickpea water into it with the remaining vinegar and whisk with an electric hand whisk until the mixture is thick and white and forms soft peaks.

3   Fold a spoonful of the acquafaba mixture into the cooled
    chocolate then add this mixture back into the remaining
    foam and fold in. Whisk briefly to bring everything together.
    Don't worry if it loses volume.

4   Spoon into a small shallow dish and scatter over the
    blueberries, followed by the pecan nuts. Chill for 2–3 hours
    or overnight. Stick 4 teaspoons into the mousse and let
    everyone dig in.

GOLDEN PAVLOVA

This mallowy meringue cake, topped with cream and fruit, is *such* a crowd-pleaser. It's also great to serve at any time of year, as you can match the fruits to the season. The idea of this flouncy crust and billowing cream filling topped with fresh fruit originates from New Zealand and is said to be named after Anna Pavlova, the Russian ballerina who visited the country during the 1920s.

The recipe requires a little cornflour to create that unmistakable mallow texture, while a spoonful of vinegar helps to stabilise the egg whites once they're whipped. This recipe is a twist on the classic. Using a combination of golden caster sugar cut with a few spoonfuls of light muscovado sugar gives it a softer toffee-like flavour, while the hazelnuts, folded into the last third of the mixture and spooned on top, give a contrast in texture and taste.

Serves 6–8

1 tsp white wine vinegar, plus a little extra
3 large egg whites
175g golden caster sugar, plus 1 tbsp to whip the cream
35g light muscovado sugar
1 tsp cornflour
25g chopped hazelnuts
300ml double cream
200g raspberries
Cocoa powder, to dust

1 Preheat the oven to 140°C/120°C fan/gas mark 1. Line a square baking sheet with baking parchment then draw an 18cm round on top, using a plate as a guide. Turn it over so the marks are underneath.

2 Take a very clean bowl and first wipe it out with a piece of kitchen paper soaked in a little vinegar – this will ensure any grease marks are wiped away. Pour the egg whites into the bowl and whisk with an electric hand whisk or in a freestanding mixer until the whites have doubled up in volume and stand in soft peaks when the beater's lifted. To test if they're ready, they should no longer be able to move around in the bowl and you should be able to turn the bowl upside down without them falling out.

3 Start to add the sugar, a tablespoon at a time, and whisk in between each addition, making sure it's properly incorporated. Continue to do this until you've added all the sugar. Add 1 tsp vinegar and the cornflour and whisk in quickly.

4 Spoon about a third of the mixture into the middle of the traced circle and smooth out to the edges.

5 Fold the hazelnuts into the remaining mixture and spoon on top, smoothing it out to the edges. Bake in the oven for 1 hour. Turn off the heat and leave to cool in the oven. You can do this up to a day ahead, just put a note on the oven to remind you it's in there.

6 To serve, whip the cream in a bowl with a tablespoon of sugar. Slide the pavlova onto a serving plate and spoon the cream on top. Scatter over the raspberries, dust with cocoa and serve.

BREAD AND BAKING

Here are three recipes for breads that can be mixed and made in minutes without any need for proving. They work on the same principle of using vinegar to help them to rise. When the vinegar is stirred into milk, the acid reacts with the raising agent (either baking powder or bicarbonate of soda) to give a light rise.

The first recipe for cornbread makes a runny batter and bakes to a sponge-like texture with a buttery flavour, spiked with chilli and thyme. Dip squares into soup – try tomato, sweet potato or butternut squash.

The third bread is a seeded soda bread, laced with a handful of oats to give it a slightly rougher texture. Serve from the oven when it's still warm. Slice and top with cream cheese, smoked salmon and sliced cornichons or a pile of creamy scrambled eggs. It's also good the next day, toasted with butter and marmalade.

All three breads freeze well. Once cool, wrap tightly in cling film and freeze for up to one month. Thaw overnight in a cool kitchen.

CHILLI AND THYME CORNBREAD

Cuts into 16 slices or squares

250ml milk
1 tbsp white wine vinegar
125g salted butter
175g self-raising flour (or self-raising gluten-free flour)
175g fine cornmeal
1 tsp salt
½–1 tsp chilli flakes
Leaves from 2–3 bushy sprigs of thyme, chopped
2 medium eggs

1   Preheat the oven to 200°C/180°C fan/gas mark 6. Line a square or round 20cm tin with baking parchment (not greaseproof or the cornbread will stick).

2   Pour the milk into a bowl, stir in the vinegar then set aside for 10 minutes. Melt the butter in a pan over a very low heat.

3   Sift the flour and cornmeal into a large bowl then stir in the salt, chilli and thyme. Make a well in the middle and crack in the eggs.

4   Pour the milk mixture into the middle of the bowl, followed by the melted butter. Mix everything together, whisking lightly to smooth out any lumps, then pour the batter into the prepared tin.

5   Bake for 30–35 minutes or until just golden on top. Turn out onto a wire rack and serve warm.

COURGETTE AND CARROT LOAF

Did you know you can bake without eggs? Swapping them for vinegar and bicarbonate of soda causes a chemical reaction (essentially carbon dioxide) that mimics the rise you get from using eggs. This recipe is a savoury offering flavoured with courgettes, carrots, chopped pecans and olive oil. It's quite moist and has a nutty flavour from the wholemeal flour, but you can by all means use plain flour if you only have that in. Serve with creamy goat's cheese and a wholesome bowl of soup to dip the slices into.

Serves 8

225g wholemeal or plain flour
1½ tsp baking powder
100g courgette, grated
75g carrot, grated
30g pecans, finely chopped
½ tsp salt
50ml olive oil
1 tbsp thick-set honey
125ml milk
½ tsp bicarbonate of soda
1 tbsp white wine vinegar

1   Preheat the oven to 200°C/180°C fan/gas mark 6. Oil and line a 450g loaf tin with baking parchment.

2   Sift the flour and baking powder into a bowl and stir in the grated courgette, carrot, pecans and salt. Make a well in the middle and pour in the oil and honey.

3 In a separate bowl, whisk together the milk, bicarbonate of soda and vinegar. Pour this into the well, too, then beat everything together until smooth. Spoon into the prepared loaf tin then level the top and bake for 1 hour to 1 hour and 30 minutes. To check it's cooked all the way through, push a skewer into the middle – it's ready whn it comes out clean.

4 Cool on a wire rack then slice and serve.

COOK'S TIP
This loaf freezes well, too. Wrap in cling film, label and freeze for up to three months. Thaw at room temperature.

SEEDED SODA BREAD

Cuts into 16 slices

250ml milk

1 tbsp white wine vinegar

350–375g plain flour (or use half plain and half wholemeal flour)

2 tsp bicarbonate of soda

1 tsp salt

1 tbsp mixed seeds

50g rolled oats

1   Preheat the oven to 210°C/190°C fan/gas mark 6½.

2   Measure the milk into a jug and stir in the vinegar. Sift the flour, bicarbonate of soda and salt into a bowl and stir in the seeds and oats.

3   Make a well in the middle and pour in the milk. Stir the wet mixture into the dry mixture really quickly – a table knife is really good for this. When you have a craggy-looking loaf, bring it together lightly with your hands, then tip onto a baking sheet.

4   Shape roughly into a round and mark a cross in the top with a knife. Bake for around 25 minutes until it is risen and golden and sounds hollow when tapped on the base. Slide onto a wire rack and leave to cool until warm (if you can bear it, that is – there's nothing nicer than the cook's perk of a small crust cut straight from a hot loaf, slathered with butter…).

PICKLES AND PRESERVES

Vinegar is essential for preserving as it helps to kill off any bacteria that could fester and grow over the traditionally long months of storing the pots. If you've never made any preserves before, these recipes are a great place to start. Each makes a small quantity so you don't need lots of tricky equipment – just a large saucepan and a spoon – nor do they need any hard-to-find ingredients.

The first three recipes make two jars – one to keep and one to give away.

RED, WHITE AND GREEN PICCALILLI

This recipe calls for a basic clear vinegar – distilled malt – and it's ready to eat as soon as you've made it. The vegetables need a short spell simmered in brine first, before they are added to a sauce that coats and preserves them. Using wholegrain mustard and white pepper isn't traditional for piccalilli, but they add a warming spiciness to the overall flavour.

Makes 2 jars - each around 250g

60g sea salt
½ cucumber, deseeded and chopped into small pieces
½ red pepper, deseeded and chopped into small pieces
175g cauliflower florets (about ½ small cauli), each floret quartered
2 large banana shallots (about 100g), chopped
275ml distilled malt vinegar
50g golden caster sugar
1 tsp each of wholegrain mustard and ground turmeric
1 tbsp plain flour
½ tsp ground white pepper

1 Pour 500ml water into a medium pan and stir in the salt. Place the pan over a low heat for around 5 minutes and stir every now and then to dissolve the salt. Add the vegetables and simmer for 5–8 minutes until tender. Drain in a colander.

2 Pour 200ml of the vinegar into a pan and add the sugar. Heat gently for a minute or two to dissolve the sugar. Mix the remaining vinegar into the mustard, turmeric, flour and white pepper. Once the sugar has dissolved, return the

vegetables to the pan and simmer over a very low heat for 8 minutes. Stir in the vinegar mixture and bring to a simmer. Cook for a further 2 minutes.

3 Sterilise two jars (see below) and divide the mixture between them. Seal and label each, including the date on which they were made. Store, unopened, in a cool dark cupboard for up to three months. Once opened, store in a cool, dry place and use within two to three weeks.

TO STERILISE JARS...

You can sterilise jars in the oven, but there is a quicker way when you only have a small number to do. First make sure the jars are clean, so wash them in hot soapy water then rinse well. Rest the jars on the bridge between a double sink or on a draining board, along with the lids, and pour boiling water into each one, making sure it flows over the side. Using rubber gloves, pour the water away (or into the washing-up bowl) and fill the jars with your ingredients. Tip the water out of the lids, give them a shake dry and use them to seal the jars.

PICKLED PEARS WITH STAR ANISE AND GINGER

Spicy ginger and the aromatic, aniseed-tasting star anise brings lots of flavour to this pickled pear recipe which calls for just five ingredients. Cider vinegar is used here, which gives the pickling juice a pleasing fruity note. These pears are a great partner to cold ham or hot roast pork, or you can slice the pieces thinly and arrange them on top of chunks of thick toast spread first with ricotta or mascarpone cheese. Choose firm, slightly unripe pears for this so they have a good acidity and don't become too soft during cooking.

Makes 2 jars – each around 275g

3 pears (around 500g)
10g fresh root ginger, peeled and cut into matchsticks
2 star anise
200ml cider vinegar
175g golden granulated sugar

1   Start by peeling the pears, then slice each through the middle, then in half again and remove the core and the calex at the bottom. Slice each quarter lengthways into two or three pieces. Put in a pan with the ginger and star anise. Pour in enough cold water to just cover, then put a lid on the pan. Bring to a simmer and cook for 10 minutes until tender. Drain the pears through a colander.

2   Pour the vinegar and sugar into the same pan (no need to wash). Heat gently for a few minutes to dissolve the sugar.

3   Return the pears to the pan, then cover and simmer over a very low heat in the syrup until they're very tender – around 10 minutes – and look almost translucent.

4   Spoon the pieces of pear, ginger and star anise equally into two clean sterilised jars (see box on page 157). Put the pan back on the heat and bring the liquid to the boil. Simmer for 5 minutes until it thickens. Divide the reduced syrup between the two jars. Seal and leave in a dark place for a week before serving. Once opened, store in the fridge and use within a month.

SPICED PLUMS WITH CINNAMON, JUNIPER AND BLACK PEPPER

You can make these sweet and sharp plums in around half an hour and you only need to wait a week for them to mature before eating. The red wine vinegar contributes that all-important acidity while the heavy-with-scent spices stop the finished pickle from tasting too sweet. Try with a mouth-tingling Cheddar – the sort where you can taste the salt crystals breaking through – or a creamy blue such as Gorgonzola.

Makes 2 jars (each around 335g)

275ml red wine vinegar
150g demerara sugar
2 short cinnamon sticks
1 tsp juniper berries
1 tsp black peppercorns
400g plums, halved and stoned

1   Pour the vinegar into a pan and add the sugar, cinnamon and spices. Heat gently and stir occasionally to dissolve the sugar. Bring up to the boil then add the plums. Cover the pan with a lid and simmer for 5 minutes to soften the fruit.

2   Sterilise two jars (see box on page 157) then divide the fruit and spices between them. Simmer the liquid left in the pan for around 6 minutes until thickened to a syrup. Pour equally into the two jars and seal. Store in a cool dry place for one week before enjoying. Once opened, keep in the fridge and eat within a month.

SUPER-QUICK BOWL OF CHUTNEY

This sharp and fruity chutney can be ready in half an hour and is a particularly good recipe for Christmas time. It's made up mainly of store-cupboard ingredients and mixes both red wine vinegar and balsamic vinegar to bring a sharp yet rich taste at the end. If you don't have any dried apricots in, try dates or figs instead. They're much sweeter, though, so use just half the quantity.

This isn't matured like a regular preserve so it is still a little sharp around the edges, but it's great with home-baked ham, pork pies and a good mature cheese that's always hanging around at that time of year.

Makes a generous bowlful

2 tbsp olive oil
1 small red onion, chopped
1 Bramley apple, peeled, cored and chopped
6 dried apricots, chopped
50ml red wine vinegar
25ml balsamic vinegar
75g light soft brown sugar

1   Heat the oil in a medium frying pan and stir in the onion. Season well and cook over a low heat for 4–5 minutes until just golden and softened.

2 Stir in the apple and apricots then pour in both types of vinegar and the light soft brown sugar. Season again and stir to dissolve the sugar. Once the sugar has dissolved, cover the pan with a lid and simmer for 12–15 minutes over a low heat.

3 Mash the apples down with the back of a spoon every now and then. Once cooked, there should still be a little liquid in the pan, which will set as it cools. Spoon into a bowl and leave to cool before serving.

INDEX

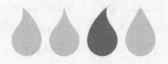